Epidemiology of Sleep
Age, Gender, and Ethnicity

Epidemiology of Sleep
Age, Gender, and Ethnicity

Kenneth L. Lichstein
H. Heith Durrence
Brant W. Riedel
Daniel J. Taylor
University of Memphis

Andrew J. Bush
University of Tennessee

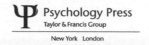

Psychology Press
Taylor & Francis Group

New York   London

First published by

Lawrence Erlbaum Associates, Inc., Publishers
10 Industrial Avenue
Mahwah, New Jersey 07430

This edition published 2012 by Psychology Press

Psychology Press   Psychology Press
Taylor & Francis Group   Taylor & Francis Group
711 Third Avenue   27 Church Road
New York, NY 10017   Hove East Sussex BN3 2FA

Cover design by Sean Sciarrone

Library of Congress Cataloging-in-Publication Data

Epidemiology of sleep : age, gender, and ethnicity / Kenneth L.
Lichstein ... [et al.]
   p. cm.
Includes bibliographical references and index.
ISBN 0-8058-4079-6 (cloth : alk. paper)
ISBN 0-8058-4080-X (pbk. : alk. paper)

RC548.E65 2004
616.8'4982—dc22   2004043440
                                                   CIP

To Harry,
my life partner.
ALF

To my mother,
who instilled in me the will to succeed and the desire to learn.
HHD

To Karen, Zach, and Katie.
BWK

To Ronald, Johnny, Lilly, Jeanie, Lottie, Joey, Eddie,
and Annette. Thanks for the love and support.
DIT

To Robert,
who makes all things possible.
AJB

Contents

Contents

Preface

Despite the presence of some 50 published epidemiological studies on sleep, only a modest amount is known about the epidemiological distribution of insomnia and less is known about the epidemiology of normal sleep. This book is a description of yet another, but unique, epidemiological study of sleep. It is the first book devoted to this topic.

How is it that such a sizable literature does not adequately inform us of sleep? The short answer is this literature is methodologically tortured and virtually ignores the majority of people, normal sleepers. The long answer is provided in the first two chapters of this book, but may be briefly summarized here. With minor exception, the existing epidemiological literature is plagued by a host of problems, including:

- Studies employed single-point, retrospective survey methods that heighten the likelihood of obtaining biased data.
- There was a preoccupation with the prevalence of insomnia, with considerably less interest in describing the nature and characteristics of insomnia.
- Inadequate, inconsistent diagnostic criteria for insomnia were used, resulting in wildly divergent prevalence estimates.
- There was little interest in normal sleepers.

The present study collected 2 weeks of sleep diaries and daytime functioning questionnaires from 772 randomly selected residents of Memphis, TN, and adjacent communities. The sample ranged in age from 20 to 98 years old, was equally divided by men and women, and achieved ethnic diversity with about 30% African American representation. This data set created a distinctive opportunity to study insomnia and normal sleep. Some of the key characteristics of our methods include:

- Using 2 weeks of data points per participant, we achieved stable sleep estimates.
- Adopting empirically justifiable, conservative, quantitative criteria for insomnia resulted in reliable prevalence data.
- We compared multiple dimensions of sleep and daytime functioning in subtypes of insomnia, and in age, gender, and ethnic groups.
- Perhaps most importantly, we produced an archive of normal sleep distributed by age, gender, and ethnicity.

Chapter 1 provides a more detailed rational for the current study and a review of its distinctive characteristics. Chapter 2 is a comprehensive review of the existing epidemiological literature on sleep. Chapter 3 presents a detailed description of the methods of this survey. Chapters 4 and 5 present archives of normal and insomnia sleep, respectively. The quality and detail of the sleep norms presented in these two chapters are unparalleled in the literature. For the first time, there is available in depth information on the epidemiology of normal and insomnia sleep. Chapter 6 is an archive of normal and insomnia sleep among African Americans. This chapter is also unparalleled in the literature. Chapter 7 is a discussion and interpretation of the most interesting findings from chapters 4, 5, and 6.

We have no illusions that this book is the final word on the epidemiology of sleep. We do believe it is a meaningful leap forward in knowledge of sleep, but we welcome replication and refinement of our data, and we eagerly anticipate the invention of methodological advances that will harvest higher quality data in the future.

Many people and institutions made important contributions to this book. A short list of acknowledgments must begin with our gratitude to the scores of students who spent thousands of hours recruiting participants. The book profited from the constructive comments of helpful reviewers including Colin A. Espie from the University of Glasgow, Tracy Kuo from Stanford University School of Medicine, Michael L. Perlis from the Sleep Research Laboratory at the University of Rochester, and Dana Epstein from the Carl T. Hayden Medical Center in Phoenix, AZ. This research was supported by National Institute on Aging grants AG12136 and AG14738, by Methodist Healthcare of Memphis, and by the Center for

Applied Psychological Research, Department of Psychology, University of Memphis, part of the State of Tennessee's Center of Excellence Grant program. Finally, without the support and patience of Debra Riegert, Lawrence Erlbaum Associates senior editor, this book would not exist.

—*Kenneth L. Lichstein*
—*H. Heith Durrence*
—*Brant W. Riedel*
—*Daniel J. Taylor*
—*Andrew J. Bush*

1

Goals and Distinctive Characteristics of This Survey

How shall we know sleep? Since the broad adoption of polysomnography (PSG), this question is not asked often enough, and is too often answered with buoyant self-assuredness.

The scientific journey of Werner Heisenberg (Cassidy, 1992) provides some perspective on how to answer this question. Like Pavlov before him, Heisenberg was a Nobel laureate, but were that his main accomplishment, he would be lost in the oblivion of history. Pavlov achieved fame not by winning the Nobel prize for his studies of the digestive processes of dogs, but as an afterthought of that research: deriving principles of conditioning that explained the behavior of dogs and others (Windholz, 1997). Heisenberg was a German physicist, and his prize was for contributions to the theory of quantum mechanics. As part of that research program, he was frustrated in his attempts to study atomic particles because the light needed to illuminate the subject altered the path of the electrons. Thus was born Heisenberg's Uncertainty Principle: The act of measurement alters what one wishes to measure, rendering specific knowledge indeterminate.

Sleep scientists in the main are probably not very sympathetic to Heisenberg's complaint. How much error could light particles have introduced to the study of electrons compared to our routine procedures? Our standard protocol is to remove individuals from their accustomed surroundings, mount a dozen or more sets of electrodes with glue, tape, straps, clips, and the like from head to foot, and then put them to rest in an uncomfortable hospital bed. It is well established that the sleep labo-

1

ratory setting alters sleep, as shown by disturbed sleep the first night in the laboratory (i.e., first night effect; Kales & Kales, 1984) and laboratory–home recording comparisons (Edinger et al., 1997; Stepnowsky, Moore, & Dimsdale, 2003). With the ease and confidence of a stand-up comic, the sleep technician instructs the individual to sleep *naturally*. Heisenberg didn't know how good he had it.

We could prove that PSG alters sleep by comparing it to a known accurate measure of sleep, but PSG is the gold standard against which other methods of sleep assessment are judged. Considering commonplace alternatives to PSG, the worthiness of actigraphy, inferring sleep from limb inactivity, or self-report (SR) sleep is evaluated by how closely they match PSG data. Of course, the matches are never perfect and assignment of fault is in part determined by convention (i.e., because PSG is objective, it is always best) and in part by philosophy of science (e.g., greater faith is assigned SR sleep in the unperturbed natural environment because it maximizes ecological validity).

Perhaps we shall never know sleep, only representations of it blurred by intrusive and/or fuzzy measures. Certainly for the present, no method of measuring sleep spares the subject of our interest. The best we could aspire to is to choose a method whose profile of strengths and shortcomings seems to closely fit the circumstances and goals of a particular clinical or research evaluation. In these endeavors, we should be humbled by the implications of Heisenberg's admonition that at all times, the relationship between sleep data and sleep is uncertain.

GOALS OF THE PRESENT EPIDEMIOLOGICAL SURVEY

This epidemiological study relied on self-report (SR) data because we wanted to collect information on a large sample and using PSG or, to a lesser extent, actigraphy would have increased the survey cost enormously, would have placed a greater inconvenience burden on participants, causing greater difficulty in recruiting the desired sample, and would have dramatically extended the length of an already lengthy study due to the limited availability of assessment instrumentation.

SR data have the advantages of:

- Being an inexpensive, convenient source of data.
- Not altering the normal sleep setting.
- Not altering normal sleep routines.
- Being the best available measure of subjective sleep perception.

We should acknowledge disadvantages of SR data that limit the infor- mation from this survey. Foremost, SR data do not inform us of sleep stages or the presence of occult sleep disorders, most notably sleep apnea or periodic limb movements. Also, the validity of SR data rests on the in- dividual's ability to recall and estimate sleep patterns, and this process necessarily introduces measurement error.

This epidemiological study was undertaken to gain knowledge about sleep that did not previously exist. Its primary goals are summarized next.

Establish Sleep Norms

Most of what we know about normal sleep derives from small-n PSG studies. In the prototypical study conducted by Williams, Karacan, and Hursch (1974), PSG data were collected from about 10 boys and 10 girls in 3- to 4-year age segments of childhood beginning with age 3–5 years and concluding with age 16–19 years. Thereafter, about 10 men and 10 women were similarly evaluated in each age decade through decade 70–79. Although this was a landmark study and was a significant ad- vance in knowledge of how people of different ages normally sleep, its findings were based on the sleep of few individuals under artificial cir- cumstances. Other methodological faults of this study can be noted. The mechanism by which participants entered this study was unspecified, but it did not appear to be a random survey, limiting its generalizability. Presumably, all participants were Caucasian (CA) because there was no mention of ethnicity.

The present study surveyed a large sample of participants, used ran- dom selection methods, and collected 14 nights of SR sleep data. Most previous epidemiological surveys of sleep have focused on insomnia and other aspects of abnormal sleep. By using sleep diaries, this survey ob- tained the largest body of data on normal sleep ever collected.

Illuminate Age, Gender, and Ethnic Differences

There have been epidemiological surveys that compared sleep among different age groups. There have been surveys that compared sleep of men and women. There have been surveys, although few in number, that compared the sleep of different ethnic groups. This is the first sur- vey to comprehensively explore sleep across the full adult age span, gender, and ethnicity.

Acquire Detailed Information About Insomnia

Most epidemiological studies of insomnia have asked little more than, "Do you have insomnia, yes or no?" (see chap. 2). Some inquired about insomnia characteristics such as time to fall asleep and time awake during the night. The present study went well beyond this standard by collecting 2 weeks of sleep diaries. These data provide detailed description of the quantitative characteristics of the insomnia and the type of insomnia. For example, chapters 5 and 6 report on the prevalence of four types of insomnia: onset, maintenance, mixed, and combined, and how these are distributed across age, gender, and ethnicity.

Identify Daytime Correlates of Sleep

Participants completed seven questionnaires on their daytime functioning. Combining this set of data with the detailed information we collected on normal and disturbed sleep, we will be in a unique position to relate multiple aspects of sleep and daytime functioning, both within and between normal sleeping and insomnia groups. Again, these analyses will be age, gender, and ethnicity sensitive.

DISTINCTIVE METHODOLOGICAL FEATURES OF THE PRESENT EPIDEMIOLOGICAL SURVEY

The extant literature contains scores of epidemiological studies of sleep, and their methodology and findings are reviewed in chapter 2. The current epidemiological study boasts a distinctive set of methodological features, creating a rich compilation of information and elevating the confidence due our findings. Most of these methods separately appear in other studies, but this set of methods appears in no other single study.

Age and Gender Dependent Sampling

Random sampling is, of course, the hallmark of an adequate epidemiological study. However, because subpopulations are unevenly distributed, random sampling guarantees underrepresentation of some segments of the population. Thus, random sampling is likely to produce insufficient numbers of some subpopulations to permit reliable statistical analyses of these groups. Similarly, reliance on unfocused random sampling to collect cases to the criterion n ensures that some segments of the population will be oversampled. This does not compromise the statistical analyses, as does undersampling, but it is inefficient and costly.

We determined our stratified sampling needs at the outset of the study. Specifically, we estimated that if we obtained at least 50 men and 50 women from each age decade beginning with ages 20–29 and ending with the decade beginning with age 80 (no upper limit was placed on this last decade), we would have sufficient diversity and balance in gender and age to adequately analyze their association with sleep. We randomly sampled without restriction until a cell (defined as men or women within each of seven decades) was filled, and then it was closed to further sampling. Sampling continued until all 14 cells were closed.

The population of the Memphis area is equally divided between African Americans (AA) and CA, so we correctly assumed ethnicity would not have to be managed in order to obtain sufficient numbers of both groups. Our final sample permits us to study sleep across the adult life span, across gender, and across ethnicity. No other epidemiological study of sleep can conduct such analyses.

Prospective

Nearly all epidemiological studies have relied on retrospective accounts. In the prototypical study, data are collected from an interview or a questionnaire in which the participant is asked if he or she has insomnia, how long has it occurred, and so on. Before proceeding, some clarification on terminology is needed. When an individual is asked to report on his or her experience, all data are retrospective. The time frame distinguishes retrospective and prospective data. The former typically asks for an estimate covering a longer, more distant period of time, as in "How long did it typically take you to fall asleep over the past month?" compared to the latter, "How long did it take you to fall asleep last night?" Prospective data maximizes the immediacy of retrospective data. [Note that although the term *prospective* usually refers to a future event, we are using it to refer to the night just completed.]

A substantial basic and applied experimental literature on retrospective compared to prospective methodology usually shows both decreased accuracy and systematic bias associated with the former. Emotionally laden experiences weigh more heavily on recall than routine events, and momentary state at the time of recall colors the retrospective account. The preponderance of data demonstrates that retrospective accounts of clinical phenomena tend to exaggerate pathology (see reviews by Gorin & Stone, 2001; Korotitsch & Nelson-Gray, 1999; Mathews, 1997). Prospective data collection fares better than retrospective with respect to both accuracy and prejudice. When individuals report on their experience from this day forward, errors due to memory fault and bias due to one's accumulated, global dissatisfaction are minimized.

Three studies have actually compared retrospective point estimates of sleep to prospective sleep diaries (Babkoff, Weller, & Lavidor, 1996; Cragg et al., 1999; Libman, Fichten, Bailes, & Amsel, 2000). Despite the lessons of research from other domains and well-established theory, the results of these three investigations are equivocal (see Table 1.1). To summarize observed patterns, better sleep was reported on sleep diaries in three comparisons (mainly sleep onset latency), better sleep was reported on retrospective estimates five times (mainly number of awakenings during the night), and no significant differences were found three times.

The expectation of a strong bias toward reporting worse sleep on retrospective estimates was not supported. However, we do not believe this question is resolved. This small set of studies prevents adequate analyses of the influence of age, gender, emotional distress, and insomnia status on these two modes of sleep reporting. As already discussed, cognitive theory most strongly predicts that people with insomnia (PWI) would unintentionally bias their memory to recall exaggerated sleep deficits, and the weight of these three studies is not sufficient to dismiss the concern that retrospective reports serve to elaborate individuals' negativistic thinking.

Multiple Sampling Points

The matter of prospective data and multiple sampling points are intertwined. Prospective data collection permits multiple sampling points. In the present study, sleep is sampled for 14 nights to yield a mean sleep parameter. Obtaining retrospective sleep data from an interview or a questionnaire, as in most prior epidemiological studies, restricts data collection to a single sampling point.

Reliability profits from averaging across multiple measurement points compared with single-point estimates. The overriding strongest influence in this matter derives from one of the most venerable of statistical concepts, the central limit theorem (Hays, 1963). The larger is the number of sampled values, the more closely their averaged value approximates the population mean and the smaller is the error associated with the estimate. The average of 14 sleep values is a more reliable measure of

TABLE 1.1
Comparison of Retrospective Estimates of Sleep and Sleep Diaries

Study and sleep variable	Age of participants[a]	Sleep status	Better sleep by diaries	Better sleep by retrospective estimate	No significant difference
Babkoff et al. (1996)	Young	PNI			
SOL			X		
NWAK				X	
TST				X	
Cragg et al. (1999)	Middle	PWI			
SOL			X		
NWAK				X	
WASO				X	
TST			X		
Libman et al. (2000)	Older	PNI and PWI			
SOL					X
NWAK				X	
TST					X
SE					X

Note. The sleep variables are sleep onset latency (SOL), number of awakenings during the night (NWAK), wake time after sleep onset (WASO), total sleep time (TST), and sleep efficiency percent (SE). PNI, people not having insomnia; PWI, people with insomnia.
[a] Young refers to young adults (approximate age range 20–40 years), middle refers to middle-aged adults (approximate age range 25–55 years), and older refers to old adults (approximate age range 55 and older).

a person's characteristic sleep than any one of those measures or any one summary retrospective estimate.

Single estimates are more vulnerable to one's psychological state, be it uncharacteristically gloomy or cheerful, at the moment of estimation. Deviant experiences, as in a recent, unusually bad night of insomnia, may exert disproportionate influence on point estimates. In contrast, averaging across multiple sampling points smoothes out occasional deviant occurrences and is more likely to fairly represent typical experience. Recent research suggests that 14 sampling points, that is, 2 weeks, of SR home sleep data are needed to establish stable sleep estimates for most sleep measures (Wohlgemuth, Edinger, Fins, & Sullivan, 1999). Only two other epidemiological studies of sleep collected prospective sleep data, that is, sleep diaries (Gislason, Reynisdottir, Kristbjarnarson, & Benediktsdottir, 1993; Janson et al., 1995). They both sampled within a restricted age range, and they both were limited to 1 week.

Comprehensive Evaluation of Daytime Functioning

Sleep cannot be well understood when insulated from the context of one's diurnal experience. The affairs of one's life, as in the presence of equanimity, distribution of exercise, and quality of diet, impact sleep, and our sleep experience reciprocates to help regulate daytime functioning. Profitable insight into the association between aging, gender, and ethnicity with sleep cannot proceed without knowledge of daytime experience. With equal certainty, knowledge of insomnia can advance little without relating disturbed sleep to the 24-hour experience.

The present epidemiological survey combines the most comprehensive evaluation of sleep with the most comprehensive evaluation of daytime functioning. The combination will hopefully yield a better understanding of both than has heretofore been possible.

SUMMARY CONCLUSIONS

This survey sets a new standard for the epidemiological study of sleep. We conducted a prospective, stratified, randomized epidemiological study of sleep across the adult life span. This was accomplished with a unique combination of methodological features that positions this data set to investigate novel dimensions of sleep and associated daytime functioning. We next construct a view of sleep sensitive to age, gender, and ethnicity differences. Our hope is that these data will enhance the clarity of our understanding of sleep, will more clearly define normal and abnormal sleep, will aid clinicians in their quest to treat insomnia, and will advance the study of sleep by stimulating further questions and inquiry among sleep scientists.

2

A Review
of Epidemiological Studies
# of Insomnia and Sleep

The epidemiological study of sleep has grown rapidly in the past 30 years. This growth is demonstrated by examining the publication dates of the 46 articles included in the present review (see Table 2.1). Only 2 of these articles were published in the 1970s, and 11 were published in the 1980s. In contrast, 26 of the articles were published during the 1990s, and 7 were published during the year 2000 or later. Thus, a rather sparse literature has rapidly evolved into a large data set. The present chapter reviews the methodology used to obtain existing data and summarizes current findings.

Our original intent in this chapter was to describe the epidemiology of both normal and insomnia sleep, but this goal was frustrated by the lack of normal sleep data. The extant sleep literature has focused on documenting insomnia prevalence rather than providing detailed descriptions of sleep. When detailed sleep data were collected, the typical approach was to merge people not having insomnia (PNI) and people with insomnia (PWI) data to report population estimates for sleep variables rather than providing separate estimates for PNI and PWI. We do report normal sleep characteristics in this chapter from the few studies that published such data, but in the main, this chapter reinforced our conviction that little is known about the self-report (SR) sleep of normal sleepers.

SELECTION OF ARTICLES TO REVIEW

A number of methods were used for locating sleep epidemiology articles. First, the electronic databases Medline and PsycInfo were used to iden-

9

tify potentially relevant articles. Second, the reference lists of existing epidemiology reviews were searched for relevant articles. Finally, we searched the reference list of each article that was examined for inclusion in the present review.

To be included, a study had to focus on adults and provide SR sleep data. Studies that provided data from objective sleep measures such as polysomnography (PSG) or actigraphy but no SR sleep data were excluded. We attempted to include studies that provided a representative sample of a particular community. Thus, a study had to employ a form of random selection from a population or had to attempt to survey an entire population (e.g., survey an entire community using a population registry). Investigations using a sample of convenience such as volunteers for a related research project, volunteers solicited from community advertisements, patients who visited a primary care physician during the course of the study, employees of a particular company, or individuals who belonged to a particular health maintenance organization were not included in the current review. We did include studies that deliberately oversampled particular groups (e.g., ethnic minorities) and studies that restricted their samples to a particular age or gender group. The resulting sample consisted of 46 studies. Pertinent results from one study were reported in two separate papers (Liljenberg, Almqvist, Hetta, Roos, & Agren, 1988, 1989), and therefore Table 2.1 includes 47 citations.

TYPICAL METHODOLOGY

Definition of Insomnia

Most papers in the current review used the term *insomnia* to refer to nighttime sleep difficulty. Other studies instead of using the term *insomnia* used alternative terms such as *sleep complaints* or *sleep disturbance* to refer to nighttime sleep difficulty. For the sake of consistency, in the current chapter *insomnia* is used to refer to nighttime sleep difficulty, and PWI will refer to people with nighttime sleep difficulty as defined by a particular study.

Data Collection Methods

Study characteristics are summarized in Table 2.1. The most popular data collection strategy was an in-person interview which was used by 19 investigations. The second most popular approach was a self-administered questionnaire ($n = 12$), often delivered through the mail, and a number of

TABLE 2.1
Characteristics of Studies Included in the Review and "Insomnia" Prevalence

Study	Geographical Location	Data Collection Technique	Sample Size	Age Range	Insomnia[a] Prevalence (%)
1. Ancoli-Israel & Roth, 1999 (Gallup Poll, 1991)	United States	Telephone interview	1000	≥18	9–36
2. Angst et al., 1989	Zurich, Switzerland	Interview (not clear if in-person)	457	27–28	12.9–46.4
3. Babar et al., 2000	Hawaii	Not clear	3296	71–93	32.6
4. Bixler et al., 1979	Los Angeles, CA	In-person interview	1006	18–80	32.2
5. Blazer et al., 1995	North Carolina	In-person interview	3976	≥65	26.6[b]
6. Brabbins et al., 1993	Liverpool, UK	In-person interview	1070	>65	35.0
7. Broman et al., 1996	Uppsala, Sweden	Mailed survey	396	20–64	15.3
8. Chevalier et al., 1999	Belgium, Germany, Great Britain, Ireland, Sweden	In-person interview	About 9000	≥18	4–22
9. Chiu et al., 1999	Shatin District, Hong Kong	In-person interview	1034	≥70	13.7–38.2
10. Doi et al., 1999	Japan	Mailed survey	1871	20–80	19.4

(continued on next page)

TABLE 2.1 (continued)

Study	Geographical Location	Data Collection Technique	Sample Size	Age Range	Insomnia[a] Prevalence (%)
11. Foley et al., 1995	Boston, New Haven, CT, Iowa	In-person interview	9282	≥65	28.5
12. Ford & Kamerow, 1989	Baltimore, Durham, NC, Los Angeles	In-person interview	7954	>18	10.2
13. Gallup Organization, 1995	United States	Telephone interview	1027	≥18	12–49
14. Ganguli et al., 1996	Monogahela Valley, PA	In-person interview	1050	66–97	50
15. Gislason & Almqvist, 1987	Uppsala, Sweden	Mailed survey	3201	30–69	26.7
16. Gislason et al., 1993	Reykjavik, Iceland	Mailed survey; 1-Week sleep diary	Survey: 430 Diary: 277	65–84	67.5
17. Habte-Gabr et al., 1991	Iowa	In-person interview	3097	≥65	18.7[b]
18. Henderson et al., 1995	Canberra and Queanbeyan, Australia	In-person interview	874	≥70	15.8
19. Husby et al., 1990	Tromso, Norway	Mailed survey	14,667	20–54	34.9
20. Janson et al., 1995	Iceland, Sweden, Belgium	In-person self-administered survey; 1-week sleep diary	Survey: 2202 Diary: 895	20–44	7.0[b]
21. Jean-Louis et al., 2000	San Diego, CA	In-person interview	273	40–64	20

Study	Location	Method	N	Age	Prevalence
22. Karacan et al., 1976	Alachua County, FL	Interview (not clear if in-person)	1645	≥18	13.8–44.6
23. Karacan et al., 1983	Houston, TX	In-person interview	2347	≥18	59.4
24. Kim et al., 2000	Japan	In-person interview	3030	≥20	21.4
25. Klink & Quan, 1987	Tucson, AZ	In-person self-administered survey	2187	≥18	37.8
26. Lack et al., 1988	Adelaide, Australia	Telephone interview	216	≥21	13.0–47.3
27. Leger et al., 2000	France	Mailed survey	12,778	≥18	9–73
28. Liljenberg et al., 1988 & 1989	Gavleborg and Kopparberg County, Sweden	Mailed survey	3557	30–65	1.6–4.8
29. Maggi et al., 1998	Veneto region, Italy	In-person interview	2398	≥65	14.7–47.3
30. Mellinger et al., 1985	United States	In-person interview	3161	18–79	17–35
31. Middelkoop et al., 1996	Krimpen aan de Lek, Netherlands	Mailed survey	1485	≥50	25.3[b]
32. Morgan et al., 1988	Nottinghamshire, England	In-person interview	1023	≥65	37.9
33. Newman et al., 1997	Maryland, North Carolina, Pennsylvania, Sacramento, CA	In-person self-administered survey	5201	65–100	65.0[b]

(continued on next page)

TABLE 2.1 (continued)

Study	Geographical Location	Data Collection Technique	Sample Size	Age Range	Insomnia[a] Prevalence (%)
34. NSF, 2002	United States	Telephone interview	1010	≥18	35–58
35. Ohayon, 1996	France	Telephone interview	5622	15–96	20.1
36. Ohayon, Caulet, & Guilleminault, 1997	Montreal, Canada	Telephone interview	1722	15–100	11.1–21.7
37. Ohayon, Caulet, Priest, & Guilleminault, 1997	United Kingdom	Telephone interview	4972	15–100	5.6–36.2
38. Olson, 1996	New Castle, Australia	Telephone interview	535	16–93	22.1–38.9
39. Partinen et al., 1983	Finland	Mailed survey	31,140	≥18	8.9
40. Quera-Salva et al., 1991	France	In-person interview	1003	16–91	48
41. Roberts, Shema, & Kaplan, 1999	Alameda County, CA	Not clear	2380	50–102	23.4
42. Rocha et al., 2002	Bambui, Brazil	In-person interview	1516	≥60	38.9

Study	Location	Method	N	Age	Prevalence
43. Seppala et al., 1997	Turku, Finland	Interview (not clear if in-person)	600	≥65	12–34
44. Sutton, Moldofsky, & Badley, 2001	Canada	Telephone interview	11,489	≥15	24
45. Welstein et al., 1983	San Francisco Bay Area	Telephone interview	6340	6–106	4.3–30.7
46. Weyerer & Dilling, 1991	Upper Bavaria	In-person interview	1529	≥15	0.4–28.5

[a]The definition of "insomnia" varied greatly across studies. A range of values is sometimes reported for prevalence within a study because some studies presented more than one definition of insomnia, resulting in multiple insomnia prevalence rates, and some studies included more than one geographical location and reported prevalence separately for each location. [b]For these studies, insomnia symptom types (difficulty initiating sleep, difficulty maintaining sleep, early-morning awakening) were reported separately, and no general insomnia prevalence was reported. For the table, the prevalence of the most common insomnia symptom type was used as "insomnia" prevalence.

studies opted for a telephone interview ($n = 10$). Only two studies used sleep diaries (Gislason, Reynisdottir, Kristbjarnarson, & Benediktsdottir, 1993; Janson et al., 1995). Most studies recruited a wide age range of participants, typically including young adults, middle-age adults, and older adults ($n = 29$). Several studies focused on older adults ($n = 16$), and one investigation included only 27- to 28-year-olds (Angst, Vollrath, Koch, & Dobler-Mikola, 1989). Strengths of the current literature include large sample sizes, careful attention to sample selection techniques, and sampling of diverse geographical locations. However, the current literature is not without problems.

Weaknesses of Current Literature and Methodological Concerns

Lack of Quantitative Detail in Describing Sleep.   Sleep epidemiology studies have focused on determining the prevalence of insomnia rather than quantitatively describing sleep. Nearly every study in the present review provides a prevalence estimate for insomnia, but few studies offer quantitative information on specific sleep variables such as sleep onset latency (SOL), number of awakenings during the night (NWAK), wake time after sleep onset (WASO), and total sleep time (TST).

Most investigators simply asked participants whether they do or do not experience insomnia or specific insomnia symptoms such as difficulty initiating sleep or difficulty maintaining sleep. One problem with this approach is that subjective views of what constitutes sleep disturbance can vary considerably across individuals (Fichten et al., 1995). Therefore, if quantitative measurement of specific sleep variables is absent, sleep differences found across groups (e.g., gender, age) could be due to subjective definitions of sleep disturbance rather than actual quantitative differences. Also, participants are forced into an all-or-nothing response (either you have disturbed sleep or not), a crude measure of sleep difficulty that decreases power to detect group differences and does not provide information on the severity of the problem.

Of the studies reviewed, only six provided mean values for SOL (Gislason et al., 1993; Janson et al., 1995; Liljenberg et al., 1988; Middelkoop, Smilde-van den Doel, Neven, Kamphuisen, & Springer, 1996; Morgan, Dallosso, Ebrahim, Arie, & Fentem, 1988; Seppala, Hyyppa, Impivaara, Knuts, & Sourander, 1997); three reported mean values for NWAK (Gislason et al., 1993; Janson et al., 1995; Middelkoop et al., 1996); and two provided mean values for WASO (Gislason et al., 1993; Liljenberg et al., 1988). TST was the most commonly assessed variable, with 13 studies reporting mean TST values (Angst et al., 1989; Broman, Lundh, & Hetta, 1996; Chiu et al., 1999; Gallup Organization, 1995; Ganguli, Reynolds, & Gilby, 1996; Gislason et al., 1993; Janson et al., 1995; Jean-Louis, Kripke, & Ancoli-Israel, 2000; Liljenberg et al., 1988; Middelkoop et al., 1996; National Sleep Foundation [NSF], 2002; Partinen, Kaprio, Koskenvuo, & Langinvainio, 1983; Seppala et al., 1997). Only seven investigations reported mean sleep variable values separately for age or gender groups (Broman et al., 1996; Chiu et al., 1999; Gislason et al., 1993; Liljenberg et al., 1988; Middelkoop et al., 1996; National Sleep Foundation, 2002; Seppala et al., 1997), and no study reported mean values separately for ethnic groups. Only two studies, both focusing on older adults, provided mean sleep variable values for different age by gender combinations (Middelkoop et al., 1996; Seppala et al., 1997).

There is not a single epidemiological study that provides normative data on a range of sleep variables across age, gender, and ethnic dimensions. Also, although studies have typically dichotomized individuals into either an "insomnia" or "normal" sleep category, there is a lack of data describing the differences between these two groups on specific sleep variables (e.g., SOL, WASO).

USE OF SINGLE-SAMPLING-POINT, RETROSPECTIVE ASSESSMENT

With the exception of two studies that employed sleep diaries (Gislason et al., 1993; Janson et al., 1995), investigators have relied on a single data sampling point consisting of an interview or self-administered survey where participants retrospectively report on their typical sleep. Such a method is potentially problematic. First, recall errors are a risk with retrospective reports, and there may be a tendency for retrospective reports to overestimate symptoms relative to more prospective methods of data collection such as daily sleep diaries. Babkoff, Weller, and Lavidor (1996) found that retrospective estimates of TST and NWAK were not significantly correlated with TST and NWAK values gathered from daily sleep diaries. SOL estimates were significantly correlated across retrospective reports and sleep diaries, but retrospective estimates were significantly longer (Babkoff et al., 1996). Another study observed that sleep variable values gathered from diaries were better correlated with PSG values than were retrospective reports of typical sleep (Carskadon et al., 1976).

Second, interpretation of retrospective data in the current literature is made even more problematic because most studies ($n = 29$, 63%) did not specify for participants the time period being assessed. For example, participants were asked how they "usually," "generally," or "currently" sleep. In the studies that did specify a time period, the time period varied greatly across studies (range = past week to past year). Third, single-point estimates may be unreliable because they may be unduly influenced by situational factors such as current mood or the most recent experience with the variable of interest (e.g., the previous night's sleep). A recent study indicated that daily assessment of sleep for a period of at least 1–2 weeks is necessary to obtain a stable estimate of most SR sleep variables (Wolgemuth, Edinger, Fins, & Sullivan, 1999). Only two studies reviewed in this chapter met that requirement by collecting 1 week of sleep diaries (Gislason et al., 1993; Janson et al., 1995).

Lack of a Consistent Definition of Insomnia

A serious problem is the lack of a consistent definition of insomnia across investigations. This leads to an absurd range in the estimated prevalence of insomnia across studies and makes the tasks of comparing and summarizing results across studies difficult. Definitions ranged from very inclusive to very restrictive. For example, on the inclusive end, Olson (1996) asked, "Have you had trouble sleeping?" and participants responded *no, occasionally, often*, or *every night*. In contrast, in the Liljenberg et al. (1988) investigation the definition of insomnia required the following: (a) an experience of getting too little sleep, (b) difficulty in initiating or maintaining sleep, (c) sleep latency or length of time awake during the night exceeding 30 minutes, (d) daytime sleepiness, and (e) a subjective deficit in sleep time exceeding 1 hour. Not surprisingly, there was a vast difference in the rate of "insomnia" reported in these two studies, with Olson (1996) finding that the prevalence of at least occasional insomnia was 38.9%, whereas Liljenberg et al. (1988) found a 1.6% prevalence rate for insomnia (4.8% when daytime sleepiness was excluded from the definition). Also, many studies considered difficulty falling asleep, awakenings during the night, and early-morning awakenings all to be indicators of insomnia, whereas other studies excluded awakenings during the night from their definition of insomnia (Foley et al., 1995; Maggi et al., 1998).

Insomnia Definitions Not Based on Accepted Diagnostic Systems

In general, definitions of insomnia used by studies were not consistent with the prevailing diagnostic systems, the *International Classification of Sleep Disorders* (ICSD; American Sleep Disorders Association, 1990) and the *Diagnostic and Statistical Manual of Mental Disorders* (*DSM–IV*; American Psychiatric Association, 1994). For a diagnosis of insomnia, both diagnostic systems require assessment of chronicity, documentation of daytime impairment, and ruling out other sleep disorders such as sleep apnea.

However, only 11 (24%) studies included assessment of insomnia duration, and only 5 studies required a particular duration for their definition of insomnia (Angst et al., 1989; Ford & Kamerow, 1989; Leger, Guilleminault, Dreyfus, Delahaye, & Paillard, 2000; Ohayon, Caulet, & Guilleminault, 1997; Ohayon, Caulet, Priest, & Guilleminault, 1997). Duration requirements ranged from 2 weeks to 1 month. Thus, there is limited information on the prevalence of chronic versus acute insomnia.

Similarly, only six studies required some form of daytime impairment in their definition of insomnia (Chevalier et al., 1999; Ford & Kamerow, 1989; Leger et al., 2000; Liljenberg et al., 1988; Ohayon, Caulet, Priest, & Guilleminault, 1997; Rocha et al., 2002). Two of these studies reported insomnia prevalence figures both with and without daytime impairment as a requirement. In both cases, the estimated prevalence of insomnia dropped substantially when daytime impairment was required (Leger et al., 2000: 29% to 19%; Liljenberg et al., 1988: 4.8% to 1.6%).

Only two studies provided prevalence rates for insomnia as defined by the *DSM–IV* or ICSD (Leger et al., 2000; Ohayon, Caulet, Priest, & Guilleminault, 1997). Leger et al. (2000) found that 73% of their sample reported sleep difficulty during the previous month, but only 19% of their participants met *DSM–IV* criteria for insomnia. Ohayon, Caulet, Priest, and Guilleminault, (1997) observed that 36.2% of their sample reported an insomnia symptom, and 8.7% reported an insomnia symptom plus sleep dissatisfaction. In contrast, only 3.6% of the sample satisfied criteria for a *DSM–IV* diagnosis of primary insomnia, and fewer met criteria for insomnia related to a medical condition (1.3%) or mental disorder (< 1%), or substance-induced insomnia (< 1%). Also, few participants satisfied ICSD-defined criteria for psychophysiological insomnia (2.2%), mood disorder with sleep disturbance (4.4%), or idiopathic insomnia (< 1%). Thus, insomnia prevalence rates reported in most studies in the current literature are probably substantially higher than rates that would be found using ICSD or DSM–IV criteria.

However, even if the ICSD or DSM–IV systems were used consistently across studies, assessment problems would still remain. Neither the ICSD or DSM–IV provides frequency (i.e., number of times per week) or severity (e.g., length of SOL, WASO) criteria for insomnia. Therefore, even these diagnostic systems rely heavily on individuals' subjective definitions of insomnia, rather than providing the clinician or researcher with quantitative criteria for determining the presence of insomnia.

SUMMARY OF CURRENT LITERATURE

Methodology of the Review

As already noted, the epidemiology literature has focused on documenting the prevalence of insomnia and particular insomnia symptoms rather than quantitatively describing sleep. Therefore, the present review focuses on the relationships between the prevalence of insomnia and insomnia symptoms (difficulty initiating sleep, difficulty maintaining sleep, early morning awakening), and age, gender, and ethnicity.

The relationship between insomnia complaints and daytime functioning is also investigated. When possible, the association between specific sleep variables (SOL, NWAK, WASO, TST) and age and gender is also explored. Finally, a few studies compared PWI and PNI on specific sleep variables, and results from these studies are summarized.

Mixed results were found on some variables, and therefore, when possible, we quantitatively summarized the results by providing a mean effect size for the comparison being discussed (e.g., the effect of gender on insomnia prevalence). Effect sizes (d) were calculated using a computer program that provides various methods for calculating d, depending on the information that is available from the article (e.g., prevalence rates for each group vs. no group prevalence rates but chi-square statistic and sample size; Shadish, Robinson, & Lu, 1997). Although the program allowed for estimation of effect size when articles report only that an effect is significant or nonsignificant, we chose not to use this method because it may lead to significant overestimation or underestimation of the true effect size.

For some comparisons (e.g., age differences for early morning awakening and age and gender differences for SOL), few studies provided sufficient information for calculating effect sizes. Mean effect sizes are reported only when at least five studies provided sufficient information to calculate effect sizes for a particular comparison. Also, calculating age effect sizes proved to be challenging because the age stratifications used to report results varied significantly across studies. However, investigators often stratified their data in a manner that allowed for comparisons of individuals 65 or 60 and older to individuals younger than 45 or 40 years, and therefore we compared these two age groups when calculating age effect sizes. In the following sections positive gender effect sizes indicate a higher prevalence in women versus men, and positive age effect sizes indicate a higher prevalence in older adults relative to younger adults. Negative effect sizes would suggest opposite outcomes. Cohen (1987) proposed that an effect size of .2 could be interpreted as a small effect, and effect sizes of .5 and .8 suggest medium and large effects, respectively.

Table 2.1 displays prevalence rates for insomnia, and Tables 2.2 and 2.3 display difficulty initiating sleep and difficulty maintaining sleep results. Studies reported early-morning awakening results less often, and these results are summarized in the text. Similar to insomnia, difficulty initiating sleep, and difficulty maintaining sleep results, sample prevalence rates for early-morning awakening varied substantially across studies (range = 2.3% to 32.3%). Table 2.4 summarizes results from studies reporting mean values for specific sleep variables. In Table 2.5 we synthesize results from the existing literature and present our best estimates of insomnia and insomnia symptom prevalence in the general population, among older adults, and among men and women.

Insomnia

Despite the lack of consistency of insomnia definitions across studies, two relatively consistent findings emerge. Subjective complaints of insomnia are more prevalent in women and increase with age.

Age Differences

There were 20 studies that included a wide age range and reported statistical comparisons for age, and the majority observed that insomnia increased with age (n = 12, 60%) or increased with age in men only (Ohayon, Caulet, Priest, & Guilleminault, 1997). Six studies

TABLE 2.2

Difficulty Initiating Sleep: Prevalence and Gender and Age Effects

Study	Difficulty Initiating Sleep Definition	Prevalence (%)	Gender Effects	Age Effects
1. Ancoli-Israel & Roth, 1999 ('91 Gallup Poll)	Sometimes or often have difficulty falling asleep	20.2	—[a]	—
2. Angst et al., 1989	Difficulty falling asleep	35.2	NS[b]	—
3. Babar et al., 2000[c]	Usually have trouble falling asleep	18.6	—	—
4. Bixler et al., 1979	Trouble falling asleep is a problem	14.4	W > M[d]	O > Y[e]
5. Blazer et al., 1995[c]	Trouble falling asleep	14.8	—	—
6. Brabbins et al., 1993[c]	Specific wording not given	25.2	W > M	—
7. Broman et al., 1996	Great or very great difficulty in falling asleep	4.6	NS	NS
8. Doi et al., 1999	Had trouble sleeping because you cannot get to sleep within 30 minutes, 3 or more times a week	10.6	W > M in 50–59 year olds and 80+ year olds	O > Y only in women
9. Foley et al., 1995[c]	Trouble falling asleep most of the time	19.2	—	—
10. Gallup Poll, 1995	Difficulty falling asleep very often	10.8	—	—
11. Ganguli et al., 1996[c]	(A) Sometimes or usually take a long time to fall asleep	36.7	W > M	NS

Study	Description	Prevalence (%)	Sex	Age
	(B) Usually take a long time to fall asleep	8.5	—	—
12. Gislason & Almqvist, 1987	(A) Great difficulty in falling asleep	6.9	—	Y > O
	(B) Moderate difficulty in falling asleep	14.3	—	—
13. Gislason et al., 1993[c]	Specific wording not given, but:			
	(A) Habitual = almost nightly	9.6	W > M	—
	(B) Occasional = 1–5 nights per week	14.4	W > M	—
14. Habte-Gabr et al., 1991[c]	SOL > 30 min (calculated based on usual time to bed and usual falling asleep time)	18.7	W > M	O > Y only in men
15. Henderson et al., 1995[c]	Trouble going to sleep nearly every night	11.7	—	—
16. Husby et al., 1990	Difficulty falling asleep at night	21.1	—	—
17. Jansor et al., 1995	Difficulty in getting to sleep at night at least 3 nights per week	7.0	NS	NS
18. Karacan et al., 1976	Trouble falling asleep	39.7	NS	Y > O
19. Karacan et al., 1983	Have difficulty getting to sleep at night			
	(A) Sometimes, often, or always	33.4	W > M	NS
	(B) Often or always	9.4	W > M	NS

(continued on next page)

TABLE 2.2 (continued)

Study	Difficulty Initiating Sleep Definition	Prevalence (%)	Gender Effects	Age Effects
20. Kim et al., 2000	Have difficulty falling asleep at night often or always	8.3	W > M	NS
21. Lack et al., 1988	Have difficulty falling asleep at night:			
	(A) Occasionally	31.9	—	—
	(B) Often	17.6	NS	NS
22. Leger et al., 2000	Difficulty initiating sleep at least 3 times a week	21.0	—	—
23. Liljenberg et al., 1988, 1989	Often or great or very often or great difficulty falling asleep	6.1	W > M	O > Y only in women
24. Maggi et al., 1998[c]	Often or always have trouble falling asleep	32.2	W > M	NS
25. Mellinger et al., 1985	Bothered a lot by trouble falling asleep	12.2	—	—
26. Middelkoop et al., 1996[c]	SOL > 30 min	12.8	W > M	O > Y
27. Morgan et al., 1988[c]	Problems in getting to sleep at least sometimes	67.5	W > M	NS
28. Newman et al. 1997[c]	Usually have trouble falling asleep	23.1	W > M	O > Y only in men

29. NSF, 2002	Difficulty falling asleep at least a few nights a week	25.0	W > M	Y > O
30. Ohayon, 1996	SOL > 30 min	24.4	—	—
31. Ohayon, Caulet, & Guilleminault, 1997	SOL > 30 min and identified by participant as major problem	10.3	W > M	—
32. Ohayon, Caulet, Priest, & Guilleminault, 1997	Quite or completely unsatisfied with SOL and SOL > 30 min or participant identifies SOL as a major problem	13.0	W > M	NS
33. Partinen et al., 1983	Have difficulty falling asleep	22.5	—	—
34. Quera-Salva et al., 1991	Have trouble falling asleep	27.3	—	—
35. Rocha et al., 2002[c]	Difficulty initiating sleep at least 3 times a week plus at least a little distress about the difficulty	19.7	W > M	—
36. Welstein et al., 1983	Have a hard time falling asleep	13.8	W > M	NS

[a]Indicates that no statistical comparisons were reported. In some cases, raw values were reported, but no statistical information was provided to indicate whether differences were statistically significant.

[b]NS indicates that there was no statistically significant effect.

[c]These studies focused on older adults.

[d]W > M indicates a statistically significant higher prevalence in women than in men, and M > W indicates a statistically significant difference in the opposite direction.

[e]O > Y (older greater than younger) indicates a statistically significant effect for age, with prevalence increasing with age. Y > O indicates a statistically significant effect in the opposite direction.

TABLE 2.3

Difficulty Maintaining Sleep: Prevalence and Gender and Age Effects

Study	Difficulty Maintaining Sleep Definition	Prevalence (%)	Gender Effects	Age Effects
1. Ancoli-Israel & Roth, 1999 (91 Gallup Poll)	Sometimes or very often wake up in the middle of the night	24.1	—[a]	—
2. Angst et al., 1989	Awakening at night	29.8	NS[b]	—
3. Babar et al., 2000[c]	Except to use the bathroom, usually wake up several times a night	7.7	—	—
4. Bixler et al., 1979	Waking up during the night is a problem	22.9	NS	O > Y[d]
5. Blazer et al., 1995[c]	Trouble with waking during the night	26.6	—	—
6. Brabbins et al., 1993[c]	Not specified	25.6	W > M[e]	—
7. Broman et al., 1996	Great or very great difficulty with nocturnal awakenings	7.5	NS	NS
8. Doi et al., 1999	Had trouble sleeping because you wake up in the middle of the night or early morning, 3 or more times a week	14.5	W > M in 20–29 year olds	O > Y
9. Foley et al., 1995[c]	Trouble with waking up during the night most of the time	29.7	—	—
10. Gallup Organization, 1995	(A) Very often wake up in the middle of the night	21.1	—	—

Study	Item	%	Sex	Age
	(B) Very often have difficulty falling back to sleep after waking up	12.7	—	—
11. Ganguli et al., 1996[c]	(A) Sometimes or usually wake up during the night and find it takes you a long time (more than half an hour) to go back to sleep	28.7	W > M	NS
	(B) Usually wake up during the night, etc.	5.6	—	—
12. Gislason & Almqvist, 1987	(A) Great problems of frequent awakening	7.5	—	—
	(B) Moderate problems of frequent awakening	14.9	—	O > Y
13. Gislason et al., 1993[c]	Specific wording not given, but:			
	(A) Habitual = almost nightly	33.5	—	—
	(B) Occasional = 1–5 nights per week	25.9	—	—
14. Husby, et al., 1990	Wake up frequently during the night	7.3	—	—
15. Karacan et al., 1976	Trouble staying asleep	11.0	NS	O > Y
16. Karacan et al., 1983	Wake up during the night after you have gone to sleep:			
	(A) Sometimes, often, or always	48.1	W > M	O > Y
	(B) Often or always	15.8	W > M	O > Y
17. Kim et al., 2000	Wake up during the night after you have gone to sleep often or always	15.0	NS	O > Y

(continued on next page)

TABLE 2.3 (continued)

Study	Difficulty Maintaining Sleep Definition	Prevalence (%)	Gender Effects	Age Effects
18. Lack et al., 1988	Wake up during the night for no particular reason:			
	(A) Occasionally	39.4	—	—
	(B) Often	19.9	NS	O > Y
19. Leger et al., 2000	Nocturnal awakenings, with difficulty returning to sleep, at least 3 times a week	16.0	—	—
20. Liljenberg et al., 1988, 1989	Troubled by nocturnal awakenings	8.3	NS	O > Y only in women
21. Maggi et al., 1988[c]	Often or always have trouble with waking up during the night	60.2	NS	O > Y only in men
22. Mellinger et al., 1985	Bothered a lot by trouble staying asleep or waking too early	10.7	—	—
23. Middelkoop et al., 1996[c]	Three or more nocturnal awakenings	25.3	W > M	O > Y only in men
24. Morgan et al., 1988[c]	Problems staying asleep at least sometimes	Not Given	NS	NS
25. Newman et al., 1997[c]	Usually wake up several times at night	65.0	NS	O > Y
26. NSF, 2002	Awake a lot during the night at least a few nights a week	36.0	W > M	NS

Study	Definition			
27. Ohayon, 1996	Awaken regularly all nights	30.0	—	—
28. Ohayon, Caulet, & Guilleminault, 1997	Nocturnal awakenings with great difficulty or inability to resume sleep or participant identifies difficulty maintaining sleep as a major problem	10.8	W > M	—
29. Ohayon, Caulet, Priest, & Guilleminault, 1997	Nocturnal awakenings with great difficulty resuming sleep or participant identifies difficulty maintaining sleep as a major problem	20.8	W > M	O > Y
30. Quera-Salva et al., 1991	Have trouble staying asleep	21.0	—	—
31. Rocha et al., 2002[c]	Disrupted sleep at least 3 times a week plus at least a little distress about the difficulty	29.2	W > M	—
32. Seppala et al., 1997[c]	One or more awakenings during sleep at least 6 nights per week	74.0	NS	NS
33. Welstein et al., 1983	Awaken during the night and have trouble getting back to sleep	15.8	W > M	O > Y

[a] Indicates that no statistical comparisons were reported. In some cases, raw values were reported, but no statistical information was provided to indicate whether differences were statistically significant.

[b] NS indicates that there was no statistically significant effect.

[c] These studies focused on older adults.

[d] O > Y (older greater than younger) indicates a statistically significant effect for age, with prevalence increasing with age. Y > O indicates a statistically significant effect in the opposite direction.

[e] W > M indicates a statistically significant higher prevalence in women than in men, and M > W indicates a statistically significant difference in the opposite direction.

TABLE 2.4
Quantitative Sleep Variables: Prevalence and Gender and Age Effects

Sleep Variable/Study	Overall (Mean)	Men (Mean)	Women (Mean)	Gender Effects	Age Effects
SOL (min)					
Angst et al., 1989	—[a]	—	—	NS[b]	—
Gislason et al., 1993[c]	36.3	—	—	—	—
Janson et al., 1995	18.0	—	—	M > W[d]	Y > O[e]
Liljenberg et al., 1988, 1989	17.8	16.0	19.6	W > M	O > Y
Middelkoop et al., 1996[c]	21.5	14.0	28.0	W > M	O > Y
Morgan et al., 1988[c]	26.2	—	—	—	—
Seppala et al., 1997[c]	34.0	28.0	41.0	W > M	O > Y
NWAK					
Gislason et al., 1993[c]	1.0	1.2	0.8	M > W	—
Janson et al., 1995	1.0	—	—	W > M	O > Y
Middelkoop et al., 1996[c]	1.9	1.7	2.1	W > M	O > Y only in men
WASO (min)					
Gislason et al., 1993[c]	31.0	—	—	—	—
Liljenberg et al., 1988, 1989	68.2	48.8	87.3	W > M	O > Y
TST (h)					
Angst et al., 1989	7.6	—	—	W > M	—
Broman et al., 1996	6.8	6.7	6.8	NS	NS
Chiu et al., 1999[c]	6.4	6.6	6.3	M > W	NS
Gallup Poll, 1995	7.0	—	—	—	—
Ganguli et al., 1996[c]	7.1	—	—	—	—

Gislason et al., 1993[c]	7.3	—	—	NS	NS
Janson et al., 1995	7.5	—	—	W > M	Y > O
Jean-Louis et al., 2000	6.9	—	—	—	—
Liljenberg et al., 1988, 1989	7.0	6.9	7.0	W > M	—
Middelkoop et al., 1996[c]	7.6	7.5	7.6	NS	O > Y
NSF, 2002	6.9	6.7	7.0	W > M	O > Y
Partinen et al., 1983	7.9	—	—	—	—
Seppala et al., 1997[c]	7.8	7.8	7.7	NS	O > Y

[a]Indicates that means were not reported separately for men and women, or in the case of gender and age effects, indicates that no statistical comparisons were reported.

[b]NS indicates that there was no statistically significant effect.

[c]These studies focused on older adults.

[d]M > W indicates that the difference between men and women was statistically significant, with men having higher values. W > M indicates a statistically significant difference in the opposite direction.

[e]Y > O (younger greater than older) indicates a statistically significant decrease in the sleep variable with increasing age. O > Y indicates a statistically significant increase in the sleep variable with increasing age.

TABLE 2.5

Prevalence Estimates for Insomnia and Insomnia Symptoms by Age and Gender

	Population (%)	Older Adults (%)	Men (%)	Women (%)
Insomnia	15.3	25.2	12.4	18.2
Difficulty initiating sleep	13.4	15.4	11.4	15.4
Difficulty maintaining sleep	15.4	25.8	13.2	17.6
Early-morning awakening	12.7	15.5	11.8	13.6

found no age difference, and only one study found a higher prevalence of insomnia in younger adults (defined as "getting too little sleep"; Gislason & Almqvist, 1987). The mean age effect size for studies comparing those 65 or 60 and older with individuals 45 or 40 and younger was .27 (*SD* = .40).

Gender Differences

Of the 33 studies that reported statistical comparisons for gender, 24 (73%) found a greater insomnia prevalence in women, 1 found a greater prevalence in older women only (Bixler, Kales, Soldatos, Kales, & Healey, 1979), and 8 observed no gender difference. No study reported a greater insomnia prevalence in men. The mean gender effect size was .25 (*SD* = .12).

Insomnia Symptoms

Age Differences

Difficulty Initiating Sleep. Thirty-six studies documented the number of individuals reporting difficulty initiating sleep (see Table 2.2). Twenty-two studies included a wide age range of participants, 13 studies focused on older adults, and one study included only 27- to 28-year-olds. Mean prevalence of difficulty initiating sleep was calculated for each group of studies, using the lower prevalence rate if multiple rates were provided within one study. The prevalence of difficulty initiating sleep was slightly higher in studies focusing on older adults ($M = 21.4\%, SD = 15.3$) than in studies with a wide age range of participants ($M = 15.7\%, SD = 8.6$), but the difference was not statistically significant, $t (33) = 1.4, p = .17$.

Thirteen studies included a wide age range of participants and reported age comparisons for difficulty initiating sleep. The majority of these studies found no age difference ($n = 7$) or found that younger sleepers had more difficulty initiating sleep than older individuals ($n = 3$). Only one study found a main effect indicating that difficulty initiating sleep increased with age (Bixler et al., 1979), and two studies found that difficulty initiating sleep increased with age only in women (Doi, Minowa, Okawa, & Uchiyama, 1999; Liljenberg et al., 1989). The mean age effect size for studies comparing those 65 or 60 and older with individuals 45 or 40 and younger was .21 (*SD* = .19).

Results were mixed in the six studies that restricted their sample to older adults but still examined age effects. Half of these studies found no increase in difficulty initiating sleep with increasing age (Ganguli et al., 1996; Maggi et al., 1998; Morgan et al., 1988), and half found that difficulty initiating sleep increased with age (Middelkoop et al., 1996) or increased with age in men only (Habte-Gabr et al., 1991; Newman, Enright, Manolio, Haponik, & Wahl, 1997).

Only four studies reported age comparisons for SOL (in minutes; see Table 2.4). Three studies found that SOL increased with age (Liljenberg et al., 1989; Middelkoop et al., 1996; Seppala et al., 1997), but one found that SOL decreased with age (Janson et al., 1995).

Difficulty Maintaining Sleep. For difficulty maintaining sleep, there were 20 studies that included a wide age range of participants and 12 studies that focused on older adults (see Table 2.3). Mean prevalence of difficulty maintaining sleep was calculated for each group of studies, using the lower prevalence estimate if two estimates were provided within the same study. The studies focusing on older adults had a significantly higher prevalence of SR difficulty maintaining sleep ($M = 34.8\%$, $SD = 22.3$) than studies with a wide age range ($M = 16.4\%$, $SD = 7.8$), $t(29) = 3.4$, $p < .01$.

In the 12 studies that included a wide age range of participants and investigated age differences in difficulty maintaining sleep, there was a clear consensus that difficulty maintaining sleep increased with age. There were nine studies that found that difficulty maintaining sleep increased with age, one study that observed that difficulty maintaining sleep increased with age in women only (Liljenberg et al., 1989), and only two studies that reported no relationship between difficulty maintaining sleep and age (Broman et al., 1996; NSF, 2002). The mean age effect size for studies comparing those 65 or 60 and older with individuals 45 or 40 and younger was .39 ($SD = .13$).

Six studies restricted to older adults investigated age differences in difficulty maintaining sleep, with three studies finding no significant age difference (Ganguli et al., 1996; Morgan et al., 1988; Seppala et al., 1997), and three studies finding that difficulty maintaining sleep increased with age (Newman et al., 1997) or increased with age in men only (Maggi et al., 1998; Middelkoop et al., 1996).

Most studies just reported a significant increase in difficulty maintaining sleep with age, but a few studies reported statistical tests between age groups that indicated when the age-related increases occurred. Bixler et al. (1979) found that difficulty maintaining sleep increased from young adulthood (18 to 30) to middle adulthood (31–50) and again after age 50, and Karacan et al. (1979) observed that difficulty maintaining sleep was more prevalent in those age 40 or older than in younger adults. Two other studies did not observe a significant increase in difficulty maintaining sleep until older adulthood (Kim, Uchiyama, Okawa, Liu, & Ogihara, 2000: ≥60; Welstein, Dement, Redington, Guilleminault, & Mitler, 1983: ≥65).

Only three studies assessed NWAK or WASO (in minutes; see Table 2.4) and reported age differences. In two of the studies NWAK or WASO increased with age (Janson et al., 1995; Liljenberg et al., 1989), and in the third study NWAK increased with age in men (Middelkoop et al., 1996).

Early Morning Awakening. A total of 26 studies reported prevalence rates for early morning awakening, with 15 including a wide age range, 10 focusing on older adults, and 1 looking at 27- to 28-year-olds (Angst et al., 1989). When prevalence rates were compared across study types, a higher mean rate of early-morning awakening was found in studies focusing on older adults ($M = 16.1\%$, $SD = 9.4$) than in studies with a wider age range ($M = 11.4\%$, $SD = 5.9$), but the difference was not statistically significant, $t(23) = 1.5$, $p = .14$.

There were 14 studies that explored age differences in early-morning awakening, including 10 with a wide age range and 4 focusing on older adults. The majority of studies including a wide age range found that early-morning awakening prevalence increased with age (Bixler et al., 1979; Janson et al., 1995; Karacan et al., 1976; Karacan, Thornby, & Williams, 1983; Kim et al., 2000; Lack, Miller, & Turner, 1988), and the remaining four studies found no age difference (Broman et al., 1996; NSF, 2002; Ohayon, Caulet, Priest, & Guilleminault, 1997; Welstein et al., 1983). Only three studies provided sufficient information to determine an age effect size for early-morning awakening, and therefore no mean effect size was calculated. All studies focusing on older adults found no significant age effect (Ganguli et al., 1996; Maggi et al., 1998; Morgan et al., 1988; Newman et al., 1997).

Total Sleep Time. There were 13 studies that reported mean values for total sleep time (see Table 2.4), including 7 studies with a wide age range, 5 studies focusing on older adults, and 1 investigation looking at 27- to 28-year-olds. No significant difference in TST was found between the studies including a wide age range of participants ($M = 7.1$ h., $SD = .42$) and investigations focusing on older adults ($M = 7.2$ h., $SD = .54$), $t(10) = 0.4$, $p = .73$.

Only three studies included a wide age range and made statistical age comparisons for TST, with one finding no age effect (Broman et al., 1996) and the others finding that TST decreased with age (Janson et al., 1995) or increased with age (NSF, 2002). Four studies focusing on older adults made age comparisons for TST, with two finding that TST increased with age (Middelkoop et al., 1996; Seppala et al., 1997) and two observing no significant age effect (Chiu et al., 1999; Gislason et al., 1993).

Summary of Age Differences. The current literature provides strong evidence that difficulty maintaining sleep increases with age. However, the prevalence of difficulty maintaining sleep may not differ between "young old" and "old old" individuals. Studies have provided mixed results regarding when increases in difficulty maintaining sleep occur, with two studies suggesting that difficulty maintaining sleep increases from young adulthood to middle adulthood (Bixler et al., 1979; Karacan et al., 1979), and two studies indicating that difficulty maintaining sleep does not increase significantly until older adulthood (Kim et al., 2000; Welstein et al., 1983). There is modest evidence that difficulty initiating sleep and early-morning awakening also increase with age. An effect size analysis indicated a small difference in difficulty initiating sleep prevalence between those 65 or 60 and older and individuals 45 or 40 and younger, and a slight majority of studies found that early-morning awakening increased with age. Only a few studies examined age effects for TST, and they produced mixed results.

Gender Differences

Difficulty Initiating Sleep. Women reporting more difficulty initiating sleep than men was a relatively consistent finding across studies (see Table 2.2). Of the 23 studies that examined gender differences in difficulty initiating sleep, 17 found that women had a higher prevalence of difficulty initiating sleep, and no study found a higher prevalence in men. The mean gender effect size for difficulty initiating sleep was .31 ($SD = .16$). Five investigations assessed gender differences in SOL (see Table 2.4). One investigation did find that SOL was significantly longer in men (Janson et al., 1995), but three studies found that SOL was significantly longer in women (Liljenberg et al., 1988; Middelkoop et al., 1996; Seppala et al., 1997).

Difficulty Maintaining Sleep. Nine studies found a higher prevalence of difficulty maintaining sleep in women, and no investigations observed greater difficulty maintaining sleep in men (see Table 2.3). However, 11 studies found no significant difference between men and women for difficulty maintaining sleep. The mean gender effect size for difficulty maintaining sleep was .17 ($SD = .19$). Two of three studies found that women experienced a greater NWAK than men (Janson et al., 1995; Middelkoop et al., 1996), and the only study to make gender comparisons for WASO found that women spent substantially more minutes awake at night (Liljenberg et al., 1988).

Early Morning Awakening. A total of 18 studies investigated gender differences for early morning awakening, with half of the studies finding that women are more likely to have early morning awakening (Brabbins et al., 1993; Ganguli et al., 1996; Karacan et al., 1983; Maggi et al., 1998; Newman et al., 1997; NSF, 2002; Ohayon, Caulet, Priest, & Guilleminault, 1997; Rocha et al., 2002; Welstein et al., 1983) and the remaining studies observing no gender effect (Angst et al., 1989; Bixler et al., 1979; Broman et al., 1996; Janson et al., 1995; Karacan et al., 1976; Kim et al., 2000; Lack et al., 1988; Morgan et al., 1988; Ohayon, Caulet, & Guilleminault, 1997). The mean gender effect size for early morning awakening prevalence was .18 ($SD = .14$).

Total Sleep Time. Nine studies explored gender differences in TST (see Table 2.4). All of the studies that focused on older adults found no gender difference for TST (Gislason et al., 1993; Middelkoop et al., 1996; Seppala et al., 1997) or found that men had a longer TST (Chiu et al., 1999). In contrast, four of the five studies that included younger participants found that women had a longer TST (Angst et al., 1989; Janson et al., 1995; Liljenberg et al., 1988; NSF, 2002), and the remaining study found no gender difference (Broman et al., 1996).

Summary of Gender Differences. There is strong evidence that women are more likely than men to report difficulty initiating sleep. There is also evidence that the prevalence of difficulty maintaining sleep and early morning awakening is slightly higher in women, but the findings for these variables are less consistent across studies. Gender differences in TST were found mostly in studies including young and middle-age adults, with women reporting longer TST.

Ethnic Differences in Insomnia Symptoms

Only four studies reported analyses investigating ethnic differences in sleep. In studies focusing on older adults, Blazer, Hays, and Foley (1995) and Foley et al. (1995) both reported that African Americans (AA) were less likely to report sleep complaints than Caucasians (CA). AA reported lower rates of difficulty initiating sleep and difficulty maintaining sleep, with the difference being particularly pronounced for difficulty maintaining sleep (AA: 19.9%; CA: 33.8%; Blazer et al., 1995). In contrast, two studies with a wider age range of participants found evidence that AA experienced more difficulty with sleep than CA (Karacan et al., 1976, 1983). One study found that AA participants in general were more likely to report sleep difficulty (Karacan et al., 1976), and the other investigation observed that AA women were more likely to experience difficulty maintaining sleep than CA and Hispanic women (Karacan et al., 1983). Karacan et al. (1983) also found that Hispanic men were less likely to report difficulty initiating sleep and difficulty maintaining sleep than AA or CA men.

Prevalence Estimates for Insomnia and Insomnia Symptoms

We derived overall prevalence estimates for insomnia, difficulty initiating sleep, difficulty maintaining sleep, and early-morning awakening from the current literature, and these results are summarized in Table 2.5. The prevalence estimate for insomnia in the population was derived by calculating the median insomnia prevalence value for the studies that included a wide age range of participants. The median rather than the mean was used to dampen the influence of outliers. If a study reported multiple prevalence rates for any measure, the most conservative rate was used for calculations. The estimate of insomnia in older adults was calculated by using the studies that focused on older adults and other studies that reported insomnia rates for older adults. From this group of studies, a median insomnia prevalence rate was calculated for older adults.

To estimate prevalence rates by gender, we first calculated the median prevalence difference between men and women in those studies including a wide age range of participants. Second, we applied this median difference to the population insomnia prevalence rate derived previously. The median insomnia prevalence rate difference between men and women was 5.8%, and therefore, using the population prevalence figure (15.3%), we estimated that the prevalence of insomnia was 12.4% and 18.2% in men and women, respectively.

These same methods were used to calculate prevalence estimates for the three insomnia symptoms. Difficulty maintaining sleep was the most prevalent symptom, followed by difficulty initiating sleep, and early morning awakening.

Insomnia and Daytime Functioning

Over half of the studies included in the current review examined the relationship between insomnia and physical health (65%), and the majority of studies also investigated the relationship between insomnia and emotional health (63%). Every one of these studies found significantly poorer physical and emotional health in PWI relative to PNI. Insomnia was significantly related to a number of specific health problems including arthritis, bronchitis, asthma, heart disease, hypertension, diabetes, and gastroesophageal reflux (Babar et al., 2000; Gislason & Almqvist, 1987; Gislason et al., 1993; Janson et al., 1995; Maggi et al., 1998). PWI consistently reported greater depression and anxiety symptoms and stress than PNI (e.g., Ford & Kamerow, 1989; Kim et al., 2000; Mellinger, Balter, & Uhlenhuth, 1985; Quera-Salva, Goldenberg, & Guilleminault, 1991).

In other studies, PWI reported more social (Chevalier et al., 1999; Gallup Organization, 1995; Ohayon, Caulet, & Guilleminault, 1997; Roth & Ancoli-Israel, 1999) and work-related (Chevalier et al., 1999) problems and decreased cognitive functioning (Gallup, 1995; Newman et al., 1997; Roth & Ancoli-Israel, 1999). Broman et al. (1996) observed greater SR fatigue among PWI. PWI SR a higher prevalence of excessive daytime sleepiness than PNI in four studies (Ganguli et al., 1996; Gislason et al., 1993; Newman et al., 1997; NSF, 2002), and a Gallup poll indicated that PWI were more likely to fall asleep in certain daytime situations (while visiting with friends, when bored; Roth & Ancoli-Israel, 1999).

A few studies examined the relationship between daytime functioning and insomnia symptom types (difficulty initiating sleep, difficulty maintaining sleep, early-morning awakening). Five studies indicated that general psychological distress or depressive or anxiety symptoms were associated with all three insomnia symptom types (Brabbins et al., 1993; Karacan et al., 1983; Kim et al., 2000; Newman et al., 1997; Quera-Salva et al., 1991). In contrast, Bixler et al. (1979) observed that anxiety was more frequently associated with difficulty initiating sleep and difficulty maintaining sleep, whereas depression was more frequent for those with difficulty maintaining sleep and early-morning awakening. However, Gislason et al. (1993) found that anxiety was associated with difficulty initiating sleep and early-morning awakening, but not difficulty maintaining sleep.

Most studies found that health problems were associated with each insomnia symptom type (Bixler et al., 1979; Janson et al., 1995; Kim et al., 2000; Newman et al., 1997). Gislason et al. (1993) found that obstructive pulmonary diseases were significantly related to early-morning awakening but not difficulty initiating sleep or difficulty maintaining sleep. One study found that daytime sleepiness was associated with difficulty maintaining sleep and early-morning awakening but not difficulty initiating sleep (Gislason et al., 1993), whereas Newman et al. (1997) found that daytime sleepiness was associated with all three insomnia symptoms in another sample of older adults. Cognitive difficulties were significantly associated with difficulty initiating sleep in general and early-morning awakening in women, but not with difficulty maintaining sleep (Newman et al., 1997).

Four studies examined the relationship between daytime functioning and specific sleep variables. Investigators found that greater TST was associated with positive mood (NSF, 2002) and fewer depressive symptoms (Jean-Louis et al., 2000). Gislason et al. (1993) observed that habitual daytime sleepiness was significantly related to greater TST at night. In another sample, gastroesophageal reflux was associated with longer SOL and greater NWAK (Janson et al., 1995).

Relationship Between Subjective Complaints of Insomnia and Specific Sleep Variables

A few studies explored the relationship between subjective insomnia and specific sleep variables. PWI consistently reported a longer SOL (Gislason et al., 1993; Middelkoop et al., 1996; Morgan et al., 1988; Ohayon, 1996), greater NWAK (Middelkoop et al., 1996; Ohayon, 1996), reduced TST (Babar et al., 2000; Chiu et al., 1999; Gallup Organization, 1995; Gislason et al., 1993; Middelkoop et al., 1996; Ohayon, 1996; Partinen et al., 1983; Seppala et al., 1997), and greater time in bed (TIB) (Morgan et al., 1988; Seppala et al., 1997) relative to PNI.

Only three studies reported mean sleep variable values for PWI versus PNI. Two studies reported a TST difference of greater than an hour between PWI and PNI (Chiu et al., 1999: 5.6 h vs. 6.9 h; Gallup Organization, 1995: 5 h vs. 7 h). In a group of older participants, Morgan et al. (1988) found that people with frequent insomnia reported that their typical SOL was about 38 min longer than PNI (53.4 min vs. 15.6 min), and their typical TIB was approximately 19 min longer (541.8 min vs. 522.6 min). One research group compared sleep variables across people who did and did not complain of specific insomnia symptom types. Complaints of difficulty initiating sleep were associated with a longer SOL (80 min vs. 25 min), and complaints of difficulty maintaining sleep were associated with a greater NWAK (1.6 vs. 1.0) (Gislason et al., 1993). Those with early morning awakening complaints awoke an average of 1 hour earlier than those without an early morning awakening complaint.

Two studies clarified that presence of an insomnia symptom is not synonymous with general sleep dissatisfaction. Ohayon, Caulet, Priest, and Guilleminault (1997) found that 36.2% of their sample reported one or more insomnia symptoms, but less than one fourth of these participants (8.7% of the sample) reported general dissatisfaction with their sleep. Similarly, Ohayon, Caulet, and Guilleminault (1997) identified a substantial group of people who reported at least one insomnia symptom but general satisfaction with their sleep quality (10.6% of the total sample, and 49.1% of those reporting an insomnia symptom).

CHAPTER SUMMARY

The current literature indicates that sleep difficulty is a widespread public health problem, affecting approximately 15% of the adult population. These nighttime sleep difficulties were consistently associated with SR poor physical and emotional health and other daytime problems.

The existing literature also suggests that insomnia is not evenly distributed across the population. A number of studies have explored age and gender differences in subjective insomnia and difficulty initiating sleep, difficulty maintaining sleep, and early-morning awakening. In general, they have found that insomnia complaints increase with age and are more likely in women. There is strong evidence that women experience more difficulty initiating sleep, and older adults experience greater difficulty maintaining sleep. There is also some evidence that women are more prone to difficulty maintaining sleep and early-morning awakening than men, and older adults are more likely to experience difficulty initiating sleep and early-morning awakening than younger adults. Unfortunately, few studies have examined potential ethnic differences in sleep, and the contrasting results of the existing studies suggest further study in this area is warranted.

Also, few epidemiological investigations have provided information on sleep variables such as SOL, NWAK, WASO, and TST, and they have relied almost exclusively on single-sample-point, retrospective reports for collecting such data. The literature would benefit from the use of sleep diaries, which provide a prospective, multiple-sample-point approach to collecting data on sleep variables. More information is needed on the relationship between specific sleep variables and age, gender, ethnicity, and daytime functioning. Also, few epidemiology studies have reported specific sleep variable values separately for PWI versus PNI.

3

Methods of This Survey

This project began with the goal of gathering stratified cross-sectional data on sleep and accompanying daytime functioning from a random sample of the city of Memphis and surrounding community. We had a relatively specific idea of what we wanted to assess in order to obtain novel normative data in this research area. We had several key night and daytime measures selected that would allow us to evaluate the sleep of the population we intended to sample. The one crucial element missing at the onset of this project was a specific sampling method.

Some years earlier, a journal reviewer advised the first author of this book to gather some normative data to support a sleep statistic (sleep quotient; Lichstein, 1997) that the present author was advocating at the time. The reviewer further wondered why this would be a difficult task, and went on to suggest that all you needed to do was make some random calls, gather some data, and you are done. After taking roughly 3 years and using 55 different telephone interviewers to call approximately 142,000 randomly generated numbers to reach 20,000 households and recruit 1700 people, we now fully appreciate the difficulties inherent in attempting this type of study.

The decision on how to gather these data was not an easy one. Two popular methods of population data collection, face-to-face interviews and random mailings, were deemed either too costly or too inefficient. A third alternative, telephone surveys, was attractive for several reasons. Household telephone coverage has vastly improved during the past 35 years in the United States (Dillman, 1978; Groves et al., 1988), to the point that most regions have a coverage rate of 95% or better. Another important factor concerns sampling expense; cost is low relative to the face-to-face interview, and data of good quality can be obtained. The added advantage of high recruiting efficiency routinely found in these surveys was also a significant factor.

Random-digit dialing is one of several types of sampling frames commonly used for telephone surveys. This technique consists of using a list of all possible telephone numbers to generate a representative sample. By using random-digit dialing, researchers are able to generate a sample that includes both listed and unlisted telephone households, thus minimizing noncoverage bias. Ideally, the only noncovered segments of the population in a random-digit dialing study are nontelephone households.

We decided to use random-digit dialing as our sampling method for several reasons. One concerned the potential for substantial coverage bias routinely found in the directory sampling method (samples are drawn from a published list of telephone numbers). Since comparisons of listed and unlisted households show important differences on many variables such as age, ethnicity, and household income, this is not a trivial consideration (Brunner & Brunner, 1971; Fletcher & Thompson, 1974). Additionally, there is a substantial financial investment required to purchase commercial telephone lists, which are the best source for telephone directories. Although approximately 80% of all possible numbers in any given central office code (telephone prefix) are not assigned to households, this method provided the best ratio of household coverage to calling expense (or at least that was what we surmised prior to study onset).

GEOGRAPHICAL AREA SAMPLED

The Memphis metropolitan area is comprised of Fayette (2.5 % of the population in 2000), Shelby (79.0%), and Tipton (4.5%) counties in Tennessee, plus Crittenden County, Arkansas (4.5%), and Desoto County, Mississippi (9.4%) (U.S. Census Bureau, 2000). Shelby County, Tennessee, has a telephone coverage rate of 96% (national average is 94.5%). The telephone coverage rates for the surrounding counties that compose the Memphis metro area are, however, significantly lower. Since Shelby County composes the largest percentage of the overall population, we decided to restrict our sample to this area. This decision also spared us long-distance phone rates in conducting the survey.

Shelby County is composed mainly of the City of Memphis, population 650,100 people (U.S. Census Bureau, 2000). Shelby County has a population of 897,472 divided nearly equally by men, 428,645 or 47.8%, and women, 468,827 or 52.2%. The ethnic distribution is predominated by Caucasian (CA) (47.3%) and African American (AA) (48.6%). The most recent per-capita income for Shelby County was 28,828 (national average is 28,546), with an average household income of $53,436 (U.S. Census Bureau, 2000). Table 3.1 summarizes the most recent education and employment data based on the 2000 census.

RECRUITMENT PROTOCOL

In order to maximize sample design efficiency, we selected at study onset (September 1997) all valid three-digit telephone prefixes currently in use in Shelby County and paired these prefixes with randomly generated four-digit numbers. This method allowed us to adhere to random-digit dialing protocol, while minimizing the costly inefficiency associated with dialing nonworking numbers. This is a common practice utilized in random-digit dialing studies (Groves et al, 1988). Given that each 10,000-number telephone prefix is not issued specific to telephone type (i.e., any given prefix will contain a mix of business, home, cellular, and unissued phone numbers), we were unable to determine household status prior to dialing each random number. Thus the majority of our random phone calls were either nonworking or to a place of business (see the Sample Characteristics section for more information about these statistics).

The random numbers were then incorporated into calling lists (see sample calling list, Fig. 3.1). These phone lists allowed us to easily identify and track all of the calls made in the course of the study. Research assistants used the lists to call the random numbers, disqualifying businesses and organizations, while tracking the nonworking numbers encountered (i.e., wrong connections, fast busy signals, and silence). They were instructed to dial each random number until they had either made a successful phone call or dialed a number five times unsuccessfully. Successful phone calls were defined as reaching one of the following outcomes: (a) nonworking numbers, (b) business numbers, (c) individuals that agree to participate, (d) individuals that do not agree to participate, and (e) individuals that do not qualify for the study. We instructed recruiters to call only during the following time periods: (a) between 10 and 11:30 a.m., (b) between 1:30 and 4:30 p.m., and (c) between 6:30 and 8 p.m. These time periods were implemented to limit calling to the best times of day to reach potential participants while avoiding times that might inconvenience the people called: the early morning, lunchtime, and late evening hours. To ensure we reached as many people as possible, we required participants to make at least one of the maximum of five phone calls in each of the three time periods.

TABLE 3.1
Shelby County Demographic Data

Variable	Census Value
Education Data	
Less than high school	17.3%
High school diploma or equivalent	30.7%
Some college, no degree	20.7%
Associate's degree	5.8%
Bachelor's degree	17.3%
Graduate degree or higher	8.2%
Occupation Data	
White collar	62.8%
Executive and managerial	11.2%
Professional specialty	14.3%
Technical support	4.1%
Sales	12.4%
Administrative support/clerical	19.5%
Blue collar	37.2%
Services	13.1%
Protective service	2.6%
Private household service	1.0%
Production	8.3%
Machine operator	4.3%
Materials	3.6%
Handlers, cleaners and helpers	4.4%

Note. These data are from the U.S. Census Bureau (2000).

TIME: 1. 10-11:30; 2. 1:30-4:30; 3. 6:30-8.
OUTCOME: 1-no answer; 2-busy; 3-answering machine;
4-bad number; 5-business; 6-call back;
7-child answered; 8-refused; 9-rejected; 10-agreed

RA_____

ID	telephone #		Date/Time/Outcome														
			call 1			call 2			call 3			call 4			call 5		
			D	T O	D	T O		D	T O		D	T O		D	T O		M
1.	262	1396															
2.	269	4313															
3.	272	6121															
4.	274	2907															
5.	276	1557															
6.	278	6995															
7.	320	3462															
8.	321	4456															
9.	323	0524															
10.	324	1032															
11.	325	1411															
12.	327	0429															
13.	329	6217															
14.	332	1535															
15.	335	7152															
16.	344	9283															
17.	345	5781															
18.	346	2618															
19.	348	7248															
20.	353	0370															
21.	354	1005															
22.	355	7326															
23.	356	2254															
24.	357	2214															
25.	358	6100															
26.	360	9539															
27.	362	2369															
28.	363	3385															
29.	365	0528															
30.	366	7383															
31.	367	1198															

FIG. 3.1. Sample of the randomly generated telephone list used to recruit participants.

Every call was coded on the call sheet (Fig. 3.1) by recording the date in the D column, the time code (1, 2, or 3) in the T column, and the outcome of the call (coded 1–10) in the O column. Codes for time and outcome were given on the top of the call sheets. A column labeled M comprised the right most column and was checked when a data packet was sent to a participant. This column proved to be unhelpful in our record keeping and its use was discontinued early on.

When a valid household was reached, the assistant delivered a prepared script that took approximately one minute and was fashioned after recommendations in Groves et al. (1988). The script comprised identifying themselves as students from the University of Memphis who were conducting survey research of people's sleep habits and associated daytime functioning.

Because this is a random sample, recruitment eligibility criteria were minimal. There were no restrictions on the participant's gender or ethnicity. Participants must have been at least 20 years of age at the day of telephone contact and must have been able to speak and read English at approximately a seventh grade level. Age and ability to speak English could be discerned during the interview. Ability to read English was not asked for in the interview script. We relied on the self-disclosure of the participant in order to avoid potentially awkward situations. We did, however, allow people with poor reading skills to participate in the study if their spouse/partner or adult child agreed to be responsible for collecting the data from the participant (we verified their agreement over the phone). We used this exception rarely and only for older adults in the 80 and older age group. We chose not to allow both cohabitating partners to participate in the study, because we feared there would be little variability in bed-partners' sleep data. Non-cohabitating members of the same household were eligible as long as they met all previous requirements. For example, we accepted participants spanning generations in the same household, such as a child, a parent, and a grandparent. In summary, we employed minimal screening criteria in order to most broadly sample the population. We had no screening criteria with respect to the presence or absence of a sleep complaint, of a conventional sleep schedule, or of health status.

Eligible individuals were asked if they would be interested in completing a 1-hour packet of questionnaires across a 2-week period in their home. They were further told that these packets inquired about their sleep habits and associated daytime functioning and that they would be reimbursed for their time. Individuals who were accepted into the study were asked to provide a mailing address. Age, gender, and mailing address were then recorded on recruitment forms for subsequent mailing. The full version of the telephone script is included as Figure 3.2.

A study packet was then mailed to the address obtained in the initial phone interview. Initially, we called the participant at 1-month

Hello, this is <u>YOUR NAME</u>. I am a student researcher at The University of Memphis. How are you doing today mam/sir. Great, the reason I have called you is to inform you that the University of Memphis is conducting a research project and looking for people in Memphis to participate.

If you are at least 20 years old, The University of Memphis will pay you $15 (or revised amount) to participate and, in addition to this cash payment, we will enter you in a $250 raffle if you complete the project.

The project is a sleep survey. It is conducted in your home and no one will call on you, nor will you have to come to the University. We will mail you the forms to complete which we call sleep diaries. What you will do is pick a 14-day period to record basic sleep information such as the time you go to bed, the time you get up, and any time during your sleep that you wake up. At the end of the 14 day period, there are 7 forms that we ask you to complete. The entire 14-day process will take approximately an hour to complete.

Would you be interested in participating in this survey for the $15 (or revised amount) payment?

(if they say yes) Super, could you give me your name? May I ask your age sir/mam? And, could you give me the address where to mail the packet?

If you have a spouse or significant other, they would **not** be eligible to also participate, but we can accept a child, parent, or grandparent over 20 years old that **lives in the household with you**. Is there anyone else in the household who is eligible and might be interested? (If yes, then get their name and age. We can interview the second person at this time, but it may be preferable to call back.) We will call back in about a week to talk with _____(the new potential participant). What would be a good time of day to call? OK, thank you very much for your time sir/mam, and you can expect that packet to arrive within a week. I will give you a call in about 2 weeks to make sure you received the packet and answer any questions you may have.

FIG. 3.2.   Telephone script used in the study.

intervals (maximum of three calls), but changed to a 2-week, 3-month system shortly after initiating the project. Approximately 2 weeks postmailing, the initial recruiter contacted the participant. These calls consisted of verifying if they had received the packet and if they had any questions at this time. We initiated these reminder calls for two purposes: (a) to ensure that they received the packet and (b) to provide a subtle reminder to begin completing the question-naires for those who had not yet begun.

If the completed packet was not received within 3 months of the mailing date, the initial interviewer (whenever possible; some of these calls were made by graduate students due to the time lag between calls and the wide use of bachelor-level students as recruiters during school semesters) made a final reminder call. This call consisted of asking them if they were having any difficulties completing the packet, and re-minding them about the potential reimbursement. If these data were not received within another month or if at any point we were unable to contact the participant by phone, a reminder letter was sent to the mailing address on file.

Study recruitment continued until data were collected from at least 50 men and 50 women in each age group beginning with the decade of 20–29 years and ending with the decade beginning with age 80. No upper limit was placed on this last decade (see Sample Characteristics section for fur-ther information). As each age decade was filled, recruitment eligibility criteria gradually became more stringent. Indeed, the final year of the study was devoted almost entirely to recruiting males 80 years or older.

Volunteers were paid between $15 and $200 for returning the com-pleted packet. We initiated the study with a flat compensation rate of $15 for completing the packet. After the first 6 months of recruitment, we observed that the pace of older adult recruitment was lagging be-hind that of younger adults. In order to add incentive to participate, we instituted a raffle that awarded $250 to one randomly selected partici-pant at the conclusion of the study. As the survey progressed, we real-ized that we were still struggling to recruit older adults and men of all ages, so we incrementally raised the compensation level to facilitate re-cruitment of these groups. The level of compensation was incrementally graduated up to $200 to recruit the final few older adults needed to complete the cohort. Table 3.2 lists the payment distribution by age and gender of the participant. Nearly half the sample (43%) was paid $15, 31% was paid $50, and 12% was paid $150. Other amounts were paid 5% of the time or less.

TABLE 3.2
Number of Participants Receiving Different Payment Amounts
by Age Group and Gender

Age Decade and Gender	$15	$30	$50	$75	$100	$125	$150	$175	$200
20–29									
Men	18	0	34	0	0	0	0	0	0
Women	50	1	1	0	0	0	0	0	0
30–39									
Men	14	1	38	0	0	0	0	0	0
Women	68	0	0	0	0	0	0	0	0
40–49									
Men	16	3	33	0	0	0	0	0	0
Women	50	0	1	0	0	0	0	0	0
50–59									
Men	11	1	44	2	0	0	0	0	0
Women	44	0	12	1	0	0	0	0	0
60–69									
Men	8	1	23	12	0	10	1	0	0
Women	31	0	12	7	0	1	0	0	0
70–79									
Men	3	1	11	0	2	1	34	0	0
Women	14	0	24	13	4	0	2	0	0
80–89+									
Men	0	0	1	0	2	1	31	14	2
Women	2	0	7	1	2	11	24	1	0
Total	329	8	241	36	10	24	92	15	2

Note. Payment data are missing for 15 participants.

Contents of Questionnaire Packet

The questionnaire packet contained sleep diaries covering 14 days, and seven daytime functioning questionnaires. For administrative purposes, the packet also included a cover sheet with instructions, two consent forms (one to return and one for the participant's records), a university reimbursement form, and a preaddressed, postage-paid envelope for returning the packet.

Sleep-Dependent Measures

Participants were instructed to complete a sleep diary upon arising each morning for 14 days. The diary is presented in Figure 3.3. Each daily diary is a brief questionnaire asking respondents to estimate particulars of their sleep experience from the night before. These diaries additionally asked about sleep medication and alcohol consumption at bedtime. To aid respondents in completing the diary correctly, it contains a sample response column and descriptions of each diary item. The diary yielded the following sleep measures.

SOL. The time in minutes it took to fall asleep counting from the moment of sleep intent. This value was derived from item 3 on the diary.

NWAK. Count of the number of awakenings during the night. The final awakening in the morning is not counted for this measure. This value was derived from item 4 on the diary.

WASO. Wake time after sleep onset in minutes or wake time during the night. SOL and wake time in bed prior to final arising in the morning do not contribute to this measure. This value was derived from item 5 on the diary.

TST. Total sleep time in minutes or actual time slept. The participant did not record this value on the dairy. TST was computed on a worksheet (Fig. 3.4) in a series of steps. Time in bed (TIB) was first computed by subtracting arise time in the morning (diary item 7) from time entering bed (diary item 2). The sum wake time during the sleep period was computed by adding SOL, WASO, and time in bed before arising (diary item 7 minus diary item 6). TST equals TIB minus sum wake time.

SE. Sleep efficiency percent is the ratio of TST to TIB $\times 100$. It is computed with the same worksheet used for TST (Figure 3.4).

SLEEP QUESTIONNAIRE
Department of Psychology, University of Memphis

ID# _____

Please answer the following questionnaire **WHEN YOU AWAKE IN THE MORNING**. Enter yesterday's day and date and provide the information to describe your sleep the night before. Definitions explaining each line of the questionnaire are given below.

EXAMPLE

		day 1	day 2	day 3	day 4	day 5	day 6	day 7
yesterday's day ⇒ yesterday's date ⇒	TUES 10/14/97							
1. NAP (yesterday)	70							
2. BEDTIME (last night)	10:55							
3. TIME TO FALL ASLEEP	65							
4. # AWAKENINGS	4							
5. WAKE TIME (middle of night)	110							
6. FINAL WAKE-UP	6:05							
7. OUT OF BED	7:10							
8. QUALITY RATING	2							
9. BEDTIME MEDICATION (include amount & time)	Halcion 0.25 mg 10:40 pm							

ITEM DEFINITIONS

1. If you napped yesterday, enter total time napping in minutes.
2. What time did you enter bed for the purpose of going to sleep (not for reading or other activities)?
3. Counting from the time you wished to fall asleep, how many minutes did it take you to fall asleep?
4. How many times did you awaken during the night?
5. What is the total minutes you were awake during the middle of the night? This does not include time to fall asleep at the beginning of the night or awake time in bed before the final morning arising.
6. What time did you wake up for the last time this morning?
7. What time did you actually get out of bed this morning?
8. Pick one number below to indicate your overall QUALITY RATING or satisfaction with your sleep.
   1. very poor, 2. poor, 3. fair, 4. good, 5. excellent
9. List any sleep medication or alcohol taken at or near bedtime, and give the amount and time taken.

FIG. 3.3. Sleep diary used in this study. Each column is used to record one night's sleep. Two pages were used to obtain 14 sleep diaries. Copyright © 1999 by Springer Publishing Company. Adapted with permission from Lichstein, Riedel, & Means (1999).

Score sheet- total sleep time (TST) and sleep efficiency % (SE)
Epidemiology of Sleep

Subject's id_______________

Rater_________________________________ date_______________

yesterday's day ⇒ yesterday's date ⇒	day 1	day 2	day 3	day 4	day 5	day 6	day 7
time leaving bed (#7)							
- time entering bed (#2)							
total time in bed (TIB)							
time to fall asleep (#3)							
wake time (#5)							
morning wake time (#7 - #6)							
Sum wake time							
TST = TIB - Sum wake time (round to 1 dec.)							
SE = TST ÷ TIB × 100 (round to 1 dec.)							

Reliability rater______________________________ final data reliability data

FIG. 3.4. Score sheet for computing TST and SE from the sleep diary.

SQR.   This is a summary quality rating of the night's experience. The rating is recorded as item 7 of the diary, and the 5-point scale is provided in the diary under the eighth item definition.

NAP.   The time in minutes spent napping the previous day. This value was derived form item 1 on the diary.

General Information and Daytime Impairment Measures

In addition to the sleep diaries, the packet contained one investigator-developed questionnaire, a health survey, and six other well-established questionnaires: Epworth Sleepiness Scale, Stanford Sleepiness Scale, Fatigue Severity Scale, Insomnia Impact Scale, Beck Depression Inventory, and State-Trait Anxiety Inventory (Trait Scale). Participants were instructed to complete this set of questionnaires on the 14th day (last day) of recording sleep diary data. Participants were instructed to answer these questionnaires as they pertained to their functioning during the previous two weeks, in order to correspond with the sleep diary data.

Health Survey.   The health survey consists of 13 items, some of which had subparts (see Fig. 3.5). We designed this questionnaire to gather important sleep and demographic information. The questionnaire collected six kinds of information: (a) demographics (e.g., height, weight, and ethnicity), (b) sleep disorders symptoms (e.g., snoring, gasping for breath during sleep, daytime sleepiness), (c) physical health (e.g., list current illnesses, medications, and vitamins), (d) mental health (e.g., describe any mental health disorders), (e) alcohol, caffeine, and nicotine consumption, and (f) educational level. In order to elucidate any relationship between physical and/or psychological functioning and sleep, an additional question asked the participants if any physical or mental illness or medication used to treat these problems has affected their sleep.

Epworth Sleepiness Scale (ESS).   This questionnaire measures trait daytime sleepiness in everyday situations (Johns, 1991). The respondents indicate how likely they are to fall asleep in eight common, quiet daytime activities over the previous 2 weeks. As examples, "Watching TV" and "As a passenger in a car for an hour without a break" are two of the items. The ratings range from 0 (*would never doze*) to 3 (*high chance of dozing*). The possible range of scores is from 0 to 24, with increasing scores indicating increasing daytime sleepiness. The ESS has demonstrated adequate reliability and good internal consistency (Cronbach's alpha = 0.88; Johns,

<u>HEALTH SURVEY</u>

Please **PRINT** and Supply **ALL** Information

ID# _____   Height _____   Weight _____

Race _____.

1. Do you have a sleep problem?   yes or no
    If yes, describe (e.g., trouble falling asleep, long or frequent awakenings, sleep apnea):

    _____

    If yes, on average, how many nights per week do you have this problem? _____

    How long have you had this sleep problem? _____years _____months

2. Please indicate whether you or your bed partner have noticed any of the following:

    Are you a heavy snorer? yes no

    Do you have difficulty breathing or gasp for breath during sleep? yes no

    Do your legs jerk frequently during sleep or do they feel restless before sleep onset? yes no

    Do you have sleep attacks during the day or paralysis at sleep onset? yes no

    If yes to any of the questions under #2, please explain and indicate how often symptoms occur:

    _____

3. Indicate with a check mark if you have the following health problems, and put the number of years you've had each problem:

Yes Years

    ___   _____   Heart disease
    ___   _____   Cancer
    ___   _____   AIDS
    ___   _____   High blood pressure
    ___   _____   Neurological disease (ex: seizures, Parkinson's)
    ___   _____   Breathing Problems (ex: asthma, emphysema)
    ___   _____   Urinary problems (ex: kidney disease, prostate problems)
    ___   _____   Diabetes
    ___   _____   Chronic Pain (ex: arthritis, back pain, migraines)
    ___   _____   Gastrointestinal (ex: stomach, irritable bowels, ulcers)

4. Please list any mental health disorders you have and the number of years you've had the disorder(s)

_____
_____

5. List any other health problems you have (and the number of years you've had the problem).

_____

6. Medical and mental health disorders may disrupt sleep. Medication may also disturb sleep. Please list any
disorder or medication that affects your sleep and describe how it affects sleep.

FIG. 3.5.   Homemade health survey used in the study.   *(continued on next page)*

7. List ALL **medications** taken within the past month, the frequency with which they are taken (e.g., daily, 3 times a day, weekly), time of day, and the purpose of the medication.

     Medicine   Frequency   Time of Day   Purpose

a. _____

b. _____

c. _____

d. _____

e. _____

f. _____

g. _____

8. List ALL **vitamins** taken within the past month, the frequency with which they are taken (e.g., daily, 3 times a day, weekly), time of day, and the purpose of the medication

     Vitamin   Frequency   Time of Day   Purpose

a. _____

b. _____

c. _____

d. _____

9. On average, how many alcoholic drinks do you drink per week? _____

10. On average, how many cigarettes do you smoke per day? _____

11. On average, how many caffeinated drinks do you have per day? _____

12. What is your highest level of education? _____

13. If you have a spouse, what is his or her highest level of education? _____

FIG. 3.5.   (*continued*)

1991). The ESS has also successfully discriminated among patients known to differ in sleepiness levels. The ESS significantly correlates with an objective measure of daytime sleepiness, the multiple sleep latency test, between rho $= -.42$ and $r = -.51$ (Johns, 1991, 1994).

Stanford Sleepiness Scale (SSS).   The SSS was originally designed to measure state sleepiness (Hoddes, Zarcone, Smythe, Phillips, & Dement, 1973). Respondents are instructed to select a level on a 7-point scale ranging from 1 corresponding to low sleepiness to 7 corresponding to high sleepiness (see Fig. 3.6) to reveal their momentary state. The SSS has since become one of the most widely used measures of state sleepiness. The SSS has been shown to be sensitive to insomnia status, usually

---

Stanford Sleepiness Scale - TYPICAL SLEEPINESS

ID# _____ Date _____

Please read all seven items below. Each describes a state of sleepiness progressing from 1 indicating not sleepy at all to 7 indicating extremely sleepy. Circle **one number** whose description best fits how sleepy you <u>usually got on a typical afternoon during the past 2 weeks</u>.

1. Feeling active and vital; alert; wide awake.

2. Functioning at a high level, but not at peak; able to concentrate.

3. Relaxed; awake; not at full alertness; responsive.

4. A little foggy; not at peak; let down.

5. Fogginess; beginning to lose interest in remaining awake; slowed down.

6. Sleepiness; prefer to be lying down; fighting sleep; woozy.

7. Almost in reverie; sleep onset soon; lost struggle to remain awake.

FIG. 3.6.   Copy of the SSS revised for this study.

producing higher sleepiness ratings for PWI (Riedel & Lichstein, 2000), produces higher sleepiness ratings in the presence of decreased sympathetic nervous system activity (Pressman & Fry, 1989), and is sensitive to manipulated sleep deprivation in normal sleepers (Herscovitch & Broughton, 1981; Hoddes et al., 1973).

However, state sleepiness does not fit well with an epidemiological survey. All of our other daytime functioning measures were completed in a single sitting at the conclusion of recording 2 weeks of sleep diaries, and we wanted this measure to conform to that procedure. Further, if we wish to relate 2 weeks of sleep to daytime sleepiness, a trait measure of sleepiness summarizing 2 weeks of experience is more useful than any particular state assessment.

We adapted this standard measure by asking participants to choose the one item that best represents their level of afternoon sleepiness over the past two weeks. Thus, the instructions given the participant converted this instrument from a state measure to a trait measure. The item content was unaltered. Figure 3.6 presents our adapted version of the SSS.

This is the first use of the SSS as a trait measure of sleepiness. At present, there are no psychometric data to address its reliability or validity.

Fatigue Severity Scale (FSS). The FSS is a 9-item questionnaire used to measure subjective severity of fatigue (Krupp, LaRocca, Muir-Nash, & Steinberg, 1989). The respondents are asked to indicate agreement with questionnaire items on a 7-point scale (1 = *strongly disagree* to 7 = *strongly agree*). Responses are averaged across the nine items, yielding a possible score range of 1 to 7. Higher scores indicate higher levels of fatigue. Sample items include "Exercise brings on my fatigue" and "Fatigue interferes with my work, family, or social life."

The questionnaire was validated on three groups: individuals diagnosed with either multiple sclerosis or systemic lupus erythematosus, and healthy adults (Krupp et al., 1989). The FSS showed high internal consistency (Cronbach's alpha = .88), clearly differentiated patients from normals (by a score ratio exceeding 2:1), and exhibited excellent test–retest reliability. Further, the FSS detected clinical progress in successfully treated subjects. Subsequent research found that the FSS taps multiple dimensions and estimates general fatigue (Schwartz et al., 1993). The FSS also appears to measure fatigue separate from daytime sleepiness (Lichstein, Means, Noe, & Aguillard, 1997).

Insomnia Impact Scale (IIS). The IIS (Hoelscher, Ware, & Bond, 1993) is the most wide-ranging index of daytime functioning available in insomnia (see Fig. 3.7). The IIS has never been published so we are presenting it here. The questionnaire contains 40 negative statements about the daytime impact of sleep. These statements sample five areas of impairment: physical, cognitive, occupational, social, and emotional. Respondents rate each item on a 5-point scale to register their degree of agreement. The range of possible scores is from 40 to 200, with increasing scores indicating increasing impact of insomnia on daytime functioning. Examples of question-

INSOMNIA IMPACT SCALE

ID#_____   Date_____

For each statement, circle the number that best describes your experience or your belief during the **past 2 weeks**.

1 = strongly disagree
2 = disagree
3 = neutral
4 = agree
5 = strongly agree

1. I am more likely to catch colds and other illnesses when my sleep is disturbed.	1 2 3 4 5
2. It is impossible for me to function the next day if I get less than seven hours of sleep.	1 2 3 4 5
3. I am less coordinated on days following poor nights of sleep.	1 2 3 4 5
4. I am afraid I may die if I don't get enough sleep.	1 2 3 4 5
5. Others can tell by looking at me when I'm not sleeping well.	1 2 3 4 5
6. Poor sleepers age faster than good sleepers.	1 2 3 4 5
7. Sleep disturbance causes me to experience nausea and headaches.	1 2 3 4 5
8. Poor sleep causes me to feel very tired and fatigued.	1 2 3 4 5
9. I can't think clearly if I don't sleep well.	1 2 3 4 5
10. The most important thing to me today is that I get a good night's rest tonight.	1 2 3 4 5
11. My sleep pattern is out of control.	1 2 3 4 5
12. I am very skeptical that insomnia can be effectively treated.	1 2 3 4 5
13. My memory is greatly affected by poor sleep.	1 2 3 4 5
14. Most people underestimate the importance of sleeping well at night.	1 2 3 4 5
15. I try to "catch" some sleep whenever I can.	1 2 3 4 5
16. I'll try anything to improve my sleep.	1 2 3 4 5
17. My mind often races at night.	1 2 3 4 5
18. I wish I could nap during the day.	1 2 3 4 5
19. Poor sleep can greatly disturb family/personal relationships.	1 2 3 4 5
20. Poor sleep prevents career advancement.	1 2 3 4 5
21. Following a night of poor sleep, I am likely to cancel my social activities.	1 2 3 4 5
22. I call in sick or go in late if I slept poorly the night before.	1 2 3 4 5
23. I avoid trips if I'm not sleeping well.	1 2 3 4 5
24. I can't help feeling grouchy and irritable following a poor night of sleep.	1 2 3 4 5
25. Poor sleep can make me feel depressed.	1 2 3 4 5
26. Almost all of my current problems in life are due to my sleep pattern.	1 2 3 4 5
27. If I have problems sleeping during the night, I become very angry.	1 2 3 4 5
28. I have developed a fear of not sleeping well.	1 2 3 4 5
29. I worry about sleep during much of the day.	1 2 3 4 5
30. I start to become anxious and tense in the evening because I might not sleep well at night.	1 2 3 4 5
31. I get so upset when I can't sleep during the night that I sometimes start crying.	1 2 3 4 5
32. I'm afraid I may kill myself if I don't start getting more sleep.	1 2 3 4 5
33. I eat more when I can't sleep.	1 2 3 4 5
34. I have problems concentrating and I make foolish errors after a poor night of sleep.	1 2 3 4 5
35. I am fidgety and restless during the day if I sleep poorly at night.	1 2 3 4 5
36. I have body aches due to poor sleep.	1 2 3 4 5
37. I feel very sleepy during the day.	1 2 3 4 5
38. Poor sleep causes my eyes to feel very heavy during the day.	1 2 3 4 5
39. Poor sleep causes me to feel lazy during the day.	1 2 3 4 5
40. Poor sleep causes me to be more socially withdrawn.	1 2 3 4 5

FIG. 3.7.   Copy of the IIS.

naire items are, "Others can tell by looking at me when I'm not sleeping well" (physical); "My memory is greatly affected by poor sleep" (cognitive); "Poor sleep prevents career advancement" (occupational); "Following a night of poor sleep, I am likely to cancel my social activities" (social); and "Poor sleep can make me feel depressed" (emotional).

To test its validity, the IIS was administered to three groups: individuals with insomnia seeking treatment, college students reporting insomnia, and college students without sleep complaints (Hoelscher et al., 1993). Mean IIS scores for these three groups were 133, 117, and 101, respectively, and each of these means differed significantly from the others. Thus, the test succeeded in discriminating people with insomnia from normal sleepers, and assuming that people with insomnia seeking treatment have a more severe problem than those who do not, it was sensitive to degree of insomnia. We have recently partially replicated these results (Means, Lichstein, Epperson, & Johnson, 2000). College students complaining of insomnia scored significantly higher on the IIS ($M = 126.4$, $SD = 18.5$) than college students reporting no sleep difficulty ($M = 96.5$, $SD = 20.0$).

Beck Depression Inventory (BDI).   The BDI is a 21-item survey that measures negative cognitions, affect, and behavior that are characteristic of depression (Beck & Steer, 1987). Each item lists four successively more disturbed statements scored 0–3, and the respondent is asked to endorse one for each item. Scores range from 0 to 63, with higher scores reflecting greater depression. It is among the most widely used depression measures. Extensive reliability and validity data have been provided by Beck, Steer, and Garbin (1988). In nondepressed participants, it may measure psychological distress (Tanaka-Matsumi & Kameoka, 1986).

State-Trait Anxiety Inventory, Trait Scale, Form Y (STAI).   The STAI consists of 20 self-descriptive statements that are rated on a 4-point scale indicating how often the statement is true (Spielberger, Gorsuch, Lushene, Vagg, & Jacobs, 1983). The test includes items concerning nervousness, worrying, and tenseness, scores range from 20 to 80, and higher scores indicate increased anxiety. The STAI shows test–retest reliability exceeding .7 and reliably distinguishes patient and normal groups (Spielberger et al., 1983).

DATA QUALITY CONTROL

This project managed a large amount of information, and common procedures were used to ensure the quality of data. The main procedures were the following.

1. All questionnaire data were scored twice independently. A supervisor compared the findings and resolved discrepancies.
2. The identity of the person doing computer data entry for each case was recorded.
3. A second research assistant visually confirmed the accuracy of all raw data entered. Discrepancies were noted and resolved by a supervisor.
4. Routine statistical procedures checked for outliers and implausible values. Suspicious scores were checked against the raw data and corrected if need be.

RESEARCH ASSISTANTS

There were in total, 55 research assistants who participated in recruitment during the sampling period. These assistants consisted of a mix of bachelor- and graduate-level students (47 bachelor, 8 graduate) at the University of Memphis who were either participating in this research for course credit (51 students) or as part of their graduate assistantship (4 students). The telephone callers were predominantly CA females (33), with only 9 students overall who were not CA. Table 3.3 lists the ethnic and gender breakdown of the research assistants from the project.

Each of the research assistants underwent four hours of comprehensive training consisting of familiarization with the recruiting protocol, simulated telephone calling with the recruitment script, followed by approximately an hour of supervised (by one of the present authors) random calling. Students were given several suggestions on how to approach initial hesitancy on the part of the interviewee. These tips included: (a) assuring the participant that the project is legitimate (a key concern for older adults, given that we were offering a relatively large monetary reimbursement for a minimum of effort), (b) pointing out that they incur no obligation by allowing us to mail them a packet, and (c) reminding them of the opportunity to further science and help a scientific project. Further training in second-effort procedures was conducted if the interviewer was recruiting at an unusually low rate relative to their peers (this is an important distinction, given the age restriction present in the latter stages of the study). Students were additionally asked to fill out the questionnaire packet themselves in order to be familiar with its contents. They were then better able to address any questions concerning the packet that came up during the telephone interview.

TABLE 3.3
Number of Research Assistants by Ethnicity and Gender

	AA	CA	Other	Totals
Men	1	13	1	15
Women	6	32	2	40
Totals	7	45	3	55

TELEPHONE CALLING SUMMARY

Table 3.4 summarizes the calling history during the survey period from September 1997 through September 2000. As this table indicates, only 19,893 (14%) of the 141,887 unique random numbers called were to valid households with potential participants. Additionally, it is worth noting (particularly for anyone considering embarking on such a costly and time-consuming enterprise) that over the course of the project an

TABLE 3.4
Telephone Calling Summary

	Frequency	Percent of Households	Percent of Total Random Numbers	Average per Month (37 Months)
Valid returned packets	772	3.9%	0.54%	22.7
Returned packets	859	4.3%	0.61%	25.3
Recruits	1,769	8.9%	1.20%	52.0
Households contacted	19,893		14.02%	585.1
Invalid phone numbers[a]	121,994		85.98%	3,588.1
Total random numbers called	141,887			4,173.1
Total phone contacts	371,560			10,928.2

[a]Includes nonworking, business, and cellular telephone numbers.

estimated 371,560 separate phone calls were made. This figure includes the 141,887 unique random numbers, 227,019 additional follow-up calls to these numbers (an average of 2.6 calls per random number were made), and 2,654 reminder calls to the 1,769 participants who initially agreed to complete the questionnaire packet (an average of 1.5 calls to each recruited participant were made). The number of follow-up and reminder calls was estimated by sampling 1,500 phone numbers.

During the course of the study, 1,769 participants were recruited out of a total of 19,893 households called (8.9%). This response rate is not indicative, however, of recruiting success, due to the restriction in recruitment imposed at the midpoint of data collection. Because we restricted age by gender deciles to approximately 50 participants, a significant percentage of ineligible (due to age restrictions) households who would have agreed to participate were actually counted as misses. Indeed, by the end of the study we were rejecting nearly 99% of all households reached in an effort to recruit the last group of men at least 80 years old. This particular age by gender decile proved difficult to fill, and was the final recruitment block completed (the next slowest age decile was completed nearly 1 year earlier). We regrettably did not attempt to distinguish between people who chose not to participate in the study (a true miss), and those who would have participated, but were rejected by us (a rejected hit). A fairer estimation of response rate would then be the response rate from the prerestriction phase of the study, or 1,155 participants out of a total of 3,215 households (35.9%).

Another distinction that we erroneously did not account for concerns confirming household status of each random number. Although we are reasonably confident we adequately distinguished invalid phone numbers from households, this is not the case concerning business numbers. We were able to rule out numbers that were obviously business related, such as those answered by automated answering services, main switchers, or receptionists. We did not, however, discern whether the person we were talking to was at a business or a household. In order to determine if this was a problem in our sample, we took approximately 500 randomly selected valid telephone numbers from across the first 1.5 years of the study (pre age restriction) and used the Cole's (reverse) Directory (Cole Information Services, 1999) to verify the status of each number. From these data we determined that an estimated 4.7% of our numbers previously coded as a household were in reality business numbers. To correct our response rate, we removed 4.7% of the 3215 households we used to calculate the previous final hit rate, leaving 3,064 total households. Thus, our final adjusted sample response rate was 1155 of 3064, or 37.7%.

Of the 1,769 recruits, 859 returned their packets, representing a return rate of 48.6%. Overall, we received data from an estimated 18.3% (estimated based on prerestricted recruiting data or 48.6% × 37.7%) of the eligible households we called during the course of the study. Of the returned packets, 87 (10.1%) had either unclear or incomplete data. The incomplete data typically involved participants not completing large portions of either the sleep diaries (the reverse side was often forgotten) or one of the daytime questionnaires. In the handful of cases with unclear data, the participants completing the packet were clearly very confused, and the data were not interpretable. The final sample consisted of 772 participants with complete, accurate data.

FACTORS AFFECTING PARTICIPATION AND RETURN RATES

We incorporated a number features recommended by Dillman (1978) to maximize the response rate. Chief among these were that the logo identifying our group was prominently stamped on the outside of the envelope so the packet would not be mistaken for junk mail and discarded, we guaranteed participants confidential handling of the information they provided, and we had follow-up reminder contacts for slow responders. There were, however, a number of potent factors operating against a high response rate.

Several key factors had a strong influence on the response and return rates and the sample characteristics of this study's sample.

Age.   There is considerable evidence that elderly persons disproportionately refuse to be interviewed in telephone surveys (e.g., Cannell, Groves, Magilavy, Mathiwetz, & Miller, 1987; Groves et al., 1988; Weaver, Holmes, & Glenn, 1975). Older adults are more likely to distrust any nonpersonal correspondence over the telephone. Media reports of telephone scams taking advantage of the elderly have contributed to this distrust, making older adult recruitment more difficult than other age groups. This phone interview reluctance was a significant issue in this sample, given our age decade recruitment strategy. Since our recruitment strategy was designed to over sample older adults (which is typically under sampled in population research), we lowered our overall response rate by employing this strategy.

Education. There is evidence that lower education groups have higher nonresponse rates (Cannell et al., 1987). This is clearly a problem for the population we sampled. The state of Tennessee has proportionately lower education rates (19% of 25- to 54-year-olds are college graduates in Tennessee, 49th out of 51 [includes the District of Columbia]; national average is 28%) than not only the national average, but also for the southern region of the United States (U.S. Population Reference Bureau, 2000). The presence of large numbers of lower education adults in Shelby County likely had a negative influence on the response rate in this sample. This phenomenon also decreased the number of AA we were able to recruit, because this ethnic group lags behind other ethnic groups in education level (U.S. Population Reference Bureau, 2000).

Interviewer Characteristics. There is clear evidence for a telephone recruitment experience effect in the research literature (Groves & Fultz, 1985). The more experienced the interviewer in survey research in general, the higher the response rate is in studies of this nature. This negatively impacted our sample, because almost all of our research assistants were young and inexperienced with telephone survey research. Given our university setting and our reluctance to pay trained professionals, this seemed to be satisfactory when we began this project. Although we have not analyzed these data, we did observe that the success of most interviewers increased over time as they amassed experience.

Participant Burden. The length and difficulty of a survey are an important factor in response rate. Both temporally (surveys spanning days or weeks) and physically (surveys with lengthy questionnaires), longer surveys tend to have lower response rates (Crawford, Couper, & Lamias, 2001; Frankel & Sharp, 1981; Groves & Kahn, 1979; Mulry-Liggan, 1983). These factors, collectively known as participant or respondent burden, are a well-established contributor to response refusal (Groves et al., 1988). In our sample we had a short initial phone interview, which was used solely for soliciting participation. After this initial interview, the participant was required to complete the questionnaire packet at home. This packet took approximately 1 hour to complete across a 2-week time period. Thus we had both a temporally and physically long study, resulting in a lower response rate.

Researchers have conducted experimental studies to document respondent burden. For example, individuals interested in reducing their alcohol consumption were randomly selected to be mailed either a short or a long questionnaire to monitor their alcohol use (Cunningham, Ansara, Wild, Toneatto, & Koski-Jannes, 1999). Participants receiving the short version of the questionnaire had a response rate of 51%, whereas those receiving the long version had a rate of 22%. It is clear from this study that increasing the length of the home questionnaire greatly reduced study participation.

In another study designed to measure the burden phenomenon, a group of researchers used a Web-based design to manipulate the perceived length of the survey (Crawford et al., 2001). Participants in one condition were asked to complete a survey that they were told would take 8–10 min, whereas those in another condition were told that the same survey would take 20 min. Those in the "shorter survey" condition had a significantly better response rate (63% vs. 68%). Apparently study duration is not the only factor involved in response burden. The participant's perception of the length of the survey is also important, a factor that probably impacted the present study. Given that our questionnaire packet is daunting at first glance, it is likely that the idea of filling out data for 2 weeks coupled with the packet's appearance resulted in attrition, even though the actual length of the survey was estimated as less than 1 hour.

Brief telephone surveys routinely obtain response rates in the neighborhood of 70% (Groves et al., 1988), but this response rate will drop rapidly as respondent burden increases. It is clear that there were numerous impediments to high response rates in this sample. With these issues in mind, it is not appropriate to compare this study's overall response (37.7%) and final return (18.3%) rate with other studies unencumbered by weighty response burden. Although there are no randomly generated population studies that include 2 weeks of sleep diaries with associated daytime functioning in the literature, there are several studies that used some form of home sleep diaries. Because these studies are similar in terms of research area and sleep diary requirement, comparing their response rates to the current project would be appropriate.

Gislason et al. (1993) and Janson et al. (1995) both conducted survey research in which they asked participants to fill out home diaries. In the Janson et al. (1995) study, participants were asked to fill out 1 week of sleep diaries that were similar in format to the ones we employed. Participants were part of a young adult random sample selected from the population registers in three European cities (Reykjavik, Iceland; Uppsala, Sweden; and Gothenburg, Sweden). Participants were mailed a sleep questionnaire, and those who responded were randomly selected for the second phase of the study. The second phase consisted of completing 1 week of sleep diaries, a sleep questionnaire, and a non-sleep-related questionnaire and health measurement. Of the 1,677 randomly selected households, 895 participants returned valid data. This return rate of 53.4% is similar to the percentage of our recruited participants who returned their data (48.6%). The difference in response rates is probably due to the additional week of sleep diaries we required of our participants. Although our overall return rate (18.3%) is considerably lower than their rate, they were not recruiting participants randomly by phone. The questionnaires were mailed to known households from a government address, and they excluded older adults.

A second similar study also gathered 1 week of sleep diary data (Gislason et al., 1993). Participation in this study was restricted to older adults on the population register of Reykjavik, Iceland. The diaries and a sleep questionnaire were mailed to the participants. Of the 800 participants, 277 returned usable sleep diary data (34.6%). This percentage is again similar to our rates.

Another example from the sleep literature comes from a random survey of sleep habits (Kripke et al., 1997). Participants were called and asked to take part in a telephone interview, with 74% agreeing to the interview. Participants were then asked to complete a home interview and sleep recording. About a third of the individuals who gave telephone interviews consented to this additional burden, dropping the overall response rate to 25%.

Across these three studies (Gislason et al., 1993; Janson et al., 1995; Kripke et al., 1997) there is an unmistakable added burden associated with collecting home sleep data and corresponding reduction in participation. Although our response rate is slightly lower than those in these similar studies, we feel that the added benefit of having a random sample, an extra week of sleep data, and concomitant, multidimensional daytime functioning data outweigh the slight improvement in response rate.

In summary, although the response rates from this study are not in the range of those found in most epidemiological research, there is evidence that this is not unusual and reflects the difficulties inherent in gathering sleep diary data. Our data set is unique among all epidemiological surveys of sleep. We asked respondents distributed across the life span to collect data for 2 weeks, completing sleep diaries each morning and completing a set of seven questionnaires on the 14th day. No epidemiological study of sleep has asked as much of participants, and no epidemiological study of sleep has collected such a rich data set. But we paid the price in response rate. In our survey, 37.7% of the households reached agreed to receive the packet, but only 48.6% of the packets were returned, producing an overall response rate of 18.3%.

Epidemiological studies are valued primarily because of their ability to randomly sample the population. We maintain that our data collection procedures were immaculate, but the final sample was not. Our use of random-digit dialing ensured that we reached all segments of the community (except those without telephones), and that we gathered a sample with as little bias as possible. However, as long as individuals retain the right to refuse to participate, self-selection will always limit the final sample, and the severity of such limitations is largely a function of participant burden. There is an irrepressible trade-off between response rate and participant burden, the cost of attempting to collect a rich data set. Even with our modest response rate, we firmly believe we succeeded in sampling the community. Our sample shows good ethnic diversity and our age-sampling procedures ensured good age diversity. We find no evidence that this process resulted in heavily skewed data.

SAMPLE CHARACTERISTICS

The final sample ranged in age from 20 to 98 years. The sample was equally balanced by gender, 381 men (49.4%) and 391 women (50.6%). This distribution maps closely onto the U.S. population of men (49.1%) and women (50.9%) (U.S. Census Bureau, 2000).

The percentage of participants sampled within age deciles is as follows: 20–29 (14%), 30–39 (16%), 40–49 (14%), 50–59 (15%), 60–69 (14%), 70–79 (14%), and 80–89+ (13%). Obtaining sufficient numbers of participants in the older decades to permit sleep analyses produced divergence from the U.S. population. For example, the age range 60 and above accounted for 41% in our sample. In the U.S. population, this group represents 16.2% (U.S. Census Bureau, 2000). As this distribution demonstrates, the findings presented in this text are based on responses from a stratified, randomly selected sample that is well balanced in terms of age and gender.

The ethnic distribution was 539 CA (69.8%), 223 AA (28.9%), 7 individuals of Asian descent (0.9%), 1 individual of Hispanic descent (0.1%), and 2 individuals for whom ethnic data were missing (0.3%). The ethnic composition of our sample does not map well on the U.S. distribution: CA (69.1%), AA (12.3%), Hispanic (12.5%), and Asian (4.2%) (U.S. Census Bureau, 2000). This is due to overrepresentation of AA in our sample and underrepresentation of other ethnic groups. This distribution does, however, provide us with sufficient numbers of AA to analyze their sleep data. Table 3.5 lists age decades by ethnicity and gender in our sample. There were 33 individuals who reported being diagnosed with a non-insomnia-related sleep disorder: 17 with sleep apnea (2.2%), 6 with periodic limb movements or restless legs (0.7%), 4 with hypersomnia (0.5%), 2 with narcolepsy (0.3%), and 4 with other sleep disorders (0.5%). Chapter 5 provides an in-depth description of the presence of insomnia in our sample.

Our investigator-designed health survey asked participants about four sleep-disorder-related symptoms. From these questions, 208 reported heavy snoring (26.9%), 89 reported difficulty breathing or gasping for breath during sleep (11.5%), 173 reported that their legs jerked frequently during sleep or that they felt restless before sleep onset (22.4%), and 80 reported having sleep attacks during the day or paralysis at sleep onset (10.5%). In our sample, 416 participants reported having none of these

TABLE 3.5
Distribution of Sample N: Age, Gender, and Ethnicity

Age Decade	Whole Sample[a]			AA			CA		
	Total	Men	Women	Total[b]	Men	Women	Total[b]	Men	Women
20–29	105	53	52	41 (39%)	18	23	61 (58%)	32	29
30–39	123	54	69	47 (38%)	18	29	72 (59%)	33	39
40–49	105	54	51	34 (32%)	18	16	71 (68%)	36	35
50–59	117	59	58	32 (27%)	12	20	84 (72%)	46	38
60–69	107	55	52	27 (25%)	9	18	79 (74%)	45	34
70–79	112	54	58	16 (14%)	6	10	95 (85%)	47	48
80–89	95	49	46	24 (25%)	12	12	71 (75%)	37	34
90–98[c]	8	3	5	2 (25%)	0	2	6 (75%)	3	3
Total	772	381	391	223 (29%)	93	130	539 (70%)	279	260

[a]Whole sample statistics include Asians and Hispanics.
[b]Parentheses specify percent within decade of total sample.
[c]For most analyses, the eight participants in the 90–98 age group were included in the previous decade, termed 80–89+.

symptoms (53.9%), 224 reported one symptom only (29.0%), 83 reported two symptoms (10.8%), 36 reported 3 symptoms (4.7%), and 13 reported having all four symptoms (1.7%). In total, 356 participants (46.1%) reported having at least one sleep- disorder-related symptom.

The health survey also asked about the presence of a variety of health difficulties. Table 3.6 summarizes the health status of our sample. To interpret these data, recall that about 70% of our sample was CA and 29% AA. These ethnic proportions should hold within each category if the disease was proportionately distributed across ethnic groups. For example, in our sample, heart disease and cancer were disproportionately underrepresented in AA and high blood pressure and diabetes were overrepresented in this group. The last column of Table 3.6 presents

TABLE 3.6
Frequency of Participants Reporting Health Difficulties
by Gender and Ethnicity

Health Problem	Men	Women	Total (with relative %)	Percent of Sample
Heart disease				
AA	7	13	20 (20%)	2.6%
CA	46	30	76 (78%)	9.8%
Total	55	43	98	12.7%
Cancer				
AA	3	3	6 (14%)	0.7%
CA	23	14	37 (86%)	4.8%
Total	26	17	43	5.5%
AIDS				
AA	0	0	0 (0%)	0.0%
CA	1	0	1 (100%)	0.1%
Total	1	0	1	0.1%
High blood pressure				
AA	24	44	68 (36%)	8.8%
CA	65	58	123 (64%)	15.9%

(continued on next page)

Total	89	102	191	24.7%
Neurological disease				
AA	1	4	5 (25%)	0.7%
CA	9	6	15 (75%)	1.9%
Total	10	10	20	2.6%
Breathing problems				
AA	9	16	25 (29%)	3.2%
CA	24	35	59 (69%)	7.6%
Total	34	51	85	11.0%
Urinary problems				
AA	11	9	20 (20%)	2.6%
CA	63	18	81 (79%)	10.5%
Total	75	27	102	13.2%
Diabetes				
AA	6	15	21 (36%)	2.7%
CA	20	16	36 (62%)	4.7%
Total	27	31	58	7.5%
Chronic pain				
AA	21	39	60 (27%)	7.8%
CA	67	94	161 (73%)	20.9%
Total	89	133	222	28.8%
Gastrointestinal				
AA	6	24	30 (24%)	3.9%
CA	36	59	95 (75%)	12.3%
Total	43	83	126	16.3%

Note. The Total row includes the 10 participants not classified as CA or AA.

prevalence rates for our whole sample within ethnic groups and for all participants positive for that disease.

Finally, the health survey asks participants about the presence of mental health disorders. In our sample 53 participants reported having a mental health disorder (6.9%, 23 men, 30 women).

Because data in this study come nearly exclusively from CA and AA, findings in this text may not fairly represent other ethnic groups. Although the study is limited in this fashion, the large random sample offers a strong basis for generalizing to the population of CA and to the population of AA and for comparing the two. The same is true for age strata and gender.

4

An Archive
of Normal Sleep

Surprisingly little is known about normal sleep. Our review of the epidemiology literature on sleep (chap. 2) strongly affirms this conclusion.
The current chapter is the most detailed, comprehensive, authoritative
accounting available on how normal people sleep.

Our first task was to determine who among our 772 cases were normal
sleepers. The present authors gave careful consideration to the matter of
how to define normal sleep and arrived at a tripartite solution.

The first group defined normality as the absence of sleep disorder. We
refer to this group as a broad definition of normal sleep. From our full
sample we eliminated 137 individuals who satisfied our definition of insomnia (described in detail in chap. 5) and 33 individuals who admitted
to another sleep disorder (described in chap. 3). Because we are analyzing sleep data by ethnicity, we excluded 9 more individuals from this
group because their small numbers do not permit analysis: 7 people of
Asian descent, 1 of Hispanic descent, and 1 individual for whom ethnicity datum was missing. We were left with a final group of 593 individuals,
comprising 76.8% of the entire sample.

The justification for this group is that normal sleep includes good and
poor (subclinical) sleepers, a normally distributed range of sleep. Our
normal sleeping group includes the subgroup often referred to as noncomplaining poor sleepers (Fichten, Libman, Bailes, & Alapin, 2000).
These are individuals whose sleep satisfies quantitative criteria for insomnia but who do not identify themselves as having insomnia. The
self-perception of having insomnia is a cardinal criterion for conferring
this diagnosis (American Sleep Disorders Association, 1990). Our normal group also includes the complementary subgroup, individuals who

complain of insomnia but for whom the magnitude of their sleep disturbance does not satisfy quantitative standards (chap. 5).

The second group is normal sleep defined narrowly. We removed from
the earlier group of 593 the noncomplaining poor sleepers (120 people)
and the individuals with sleep complaints that didn't satisfy our definition of insomnia (81 people). There remained 392 pristine sleepers,
comprising 50.8% of the entire sample. This group had no sleep complaints and did not exhibit the quantitative characteristics of insomnia.
This group could be considered a clinically normal group as compared
with group 1 representing a broader statistical sampling of non-
pathological sleep. Group 1 provides a model of the normal range of
sleep and group 2 a portrait of the best sleep reasonably possible and a
snapshot of goal sleep for discontent individuals.

The entire sample, 772 people, comprises the third group. One could
argue that the normal distribution of sleep includes all members of the
population and that individuals with sleep disorders justifiably comprise
the tail of that distribution.

ANALYTICAL BOUNDARIES OF THIS CHAPTER

The analyses of this chapter focus on groups 1 and 2. We conducted no
analyses on the third group, but did include its data in the appendix to
this chapter. The appendix includes seven tables on the first group
(Appendix Tables A4.1 to A4.7), seven more on the second group (Appendix Tables A4.8 to A4.14), and seven more on the third group (Appendix Tables A4.15 to A4.21). Each table presents means and
standard deviations for seven sleep variables within an age decade
starting with decade 20 (ages 20–29) and ending with decade 80 (ages
80–89+). The precise construction of the data comprised averaging
across the 14 sleep diaries to produce 1 point value for each sleep measure per participant. Table data represent aggregating these point estimates across participants. Each table also breaks down sleep by gender
and ethnicity. These 21 tables are an archive of normal sleep, with normalcy being defined three ways.

The ethnicity factor comparing the sleep of African Americans (AA)
and Caucasians (CA) is included in the omnibus analyses in this chapter.
However, detailed analyses of this factor are reserved for chapter 6,
where we describe data on the sleep of AA reporting both normal sleep
and insomnia. We have a rich data set on the sleep of AA, the most complete ever collected. We wish to fully explore the sleep of this subgroup of

the population in one coherent section, rather than fragmenting this body of information by distributing it across two chapters.

GENERALIZABILITY OF THESE DATA: STRENGTHS AND LIMITATIONS

The appendix tables do not provide summary data collapsing across age, gender, and ethnicity. Our sampling plan was dedicated to obtaining large-scale, representative random samples within age, gender, and ethnic strata that provided adequate coverage for all strata. We implemented this plan to enable development of quality estimates of sleeping pattern parameters within strata and to permit powerful statistical tests of differences in those parameters across strata. In so doing, we intentionally oversampled some strata in terms of their relative occurrence in the United States population at large. As a result, we do not make unconditional generalizations about sleep patterns over all strata.

Specifically, summary generalizations from this data set are constrained mainly by two factors. First, the age and ethnicity characteristics of our sample are not representative of the population. Our sampling techniques obtained sufficient samples at each adult age decade to track sleep, but in so doing, the distribution of ages maps poorly onto the population. Older adults are overrepresented. Further, our sample represents a greater proportion of AA than exists nationally. Second, because sleep differences occur with age, gender, and ethnicity, aggregate statements will over- or underestimate prevalence within stratified demographic attributes unless population-derived weights are applied as is done in chapter 5 to obtain a population estimate of insomnia prevalence.

Based on the pattern of results for main and interaction effects, it would be fair to generalize sleep observations to the population for main effects when they occur in the absence of significant interactions. Interpretation limitations in this chapter (and chaps. 5 and 6) are identified as the results are presented. When such restrictions are not stated, it is our opinion that generalization to the population for our data is fair.

The strength of this survey is based on the quality of data we obtained and the diversity of ages and ethnic groups represented. Most often, conclusions should be specific to some combination of demographic attributes.

METHODS OF STATISTICAL ANALYSIS

There is great overlap in the types of statistical procedures used in this and the following two chapters. We describe them once. We have performed statistical analyses on the data, and reserve use of the word *signif-icant* for relationships that satisfy the conventional Type I error rate of .05. However, we do not want these three chapters to read with the same level of detailed statistical reporting characteristic of journal articles. That would grow tiresome in a monograph of this length. We report om-nibus statistical results, but do not report the details of follow-up and post hoc testing, even though these have been conducted.

The main statistical tools for these analytical chapters are mult-ivariate analysis of variance (MANOVA), trend analysis, and multiple regression. To conservatively manage a set of seven sleep measures, we used MANOVA as the gatekeeper procedure to protect against spuri-ous findings resulting from inflated Type I error rates that are liable to occur with multiple analyses of variance (ANOVAs). All MANOVA results used the Wilks' Λ statistic. Trend analysis was favored over post hoc pairwise comparisons to chart sleep changes over the seven de-cades of sleep. There were many such analyses and we felt determining the main trends would be more informative than a detailed account of decade to decade changes. Lastly, regression was used to investigate the association between sleep and daytime functioning within age and gender subgroups.

MANAGEMENT OF MISSING DATA

There was a small amount of missing data among key variables, the seven sleep variables and the six daytime functioning questionnaires (exclud-ing the health survey). An accounting of the occurrence of missing data is presented in Table 4.1.

Only one of the sleep variables had missing data, sleep quality rating (SQR), and this occurred with one participant. Such a small amount of sleep missing data occurred because these are mean data points derived from 14 days of sleep diaries. If a participant omitted data for a sleep vari-able on some days, we still had data on which to compute a mean. On only one occasion did a participant omit all 14 days of data for a sleep variable. Among the remaining six questionnaires, only two participants had missing data on more than one variable. In both cases the same two variables were missing, Epworth Sleepiness Scale (ESS) and Stanford Sleepiness Scale (SSS).

A total of 16 participants produced at least one missing data point on these 13 variables. In total, 18 data points were missing from a sample of 772 cases. Ordinarily, such a small amount of missing data would be ig-

TABLE 4.1
Distribution Count of Missing Data

Variable	Number of Participants Missing Data on This Variable	Percent of Data Set
Mean SQR	1	0.1
ESS	2	0.3
SSS	9	1.2
FSS	2	0.3
IIS	1	0.1
BDI	2	0.3
STAI	1	0.1

nored, but our reliance on multivariate statistics inflates the impact of missing data. In such statistics, all data for a case are discarded when there is missing data for any one variable.

We used the single imputation method of regression substitution (Shadish, Cook, & Campbell, 2002; Sinharay, Stern, & Russell, 2001). This is a middle-grade method with respect to preserving the integrity of variance for a variable. Compared to mean substitution, which underestimates variance, and the more sophisticated multiple imputation techniques, which more adequately model variance, single imputation is a reasonable compromise that takes advantage of ease of computation while moderately addressing the issue of variance among missing values. In our judgment, particularly because our missing data accounts for a tiny percentage of the sample, single imputation is a satisfactory method.

We proceeded by collecting about two dozen predictor variables: all of the sleep variables, all of the daytime functioning questionnaires, common demographics such as age, gender, and ethnicity, and other plausible predictors such as alcohol and caffeine consumption, cigarette use, pain report, and so on. All predictor variables, except the outcome variable, were entered into the multiple regression equation for each of the missing data variables. To protect against multicollinearity distortion that is likely to occur with so many predictors, we screened out variables with $R \geq .75$ (SPSS tolerance value set at .44). By this method we predicted the 18 missing data points and inserted the estimated values.

All of the regressions for the seven missing variables produced significant Rs (presented in order of ascending magnitude): ESS = .48, SSS = .51, SQR = .63, Fatigue Severity Scale (FSS) = .66, Insomnia Impact Scale (IIS) = .70, Beck Depression Inventory (BDI) = .78, and State-Trait Anxiety Inventory (STAI) = .78. All 18 imputed values were confirmed to be plausible.

BROAD NORMAL SAMPLE: SLEEP BY AGE, GENDER, AND ETHNICITY

We began with a three-factor MANOVA, 7 age decades × 2 gender × 2 ethnicity for seven sleep measures, sleep onset latency (SOL), number of awakenings during the night (NWAK), wake time after sleep onset (WASO), total sleep time (TST), sleep efficiency percent (SE), SQR, and time spent napping (NAP). The results of this analysis are summarized in Table 4.2.

We found significant main effects for our three factors, age, gender, and ethnicity, and we found one significant interaction, age × ethnicity. The MANOVA analyzes the seven sleep measures as a single set, permitting us

TABLE 4.2
Broad Normal Sample: MANOVA Results for Sleep Measures
by Age, Gender, and Ethnicity

Factor	Wilks' Λ	df	F Equivalent
Age	.75	42, 2625	3.96***
Gender	.96	7, 559	3.38**
Ethnicity	.86	7, 559	14.00***
Age × gender	.93	42, 2625	1.02
Age × ethnicity	.90	42, 2625	1.47*
Gender × ethnicity	.98	7, 559	1.62
Age × gender × ethnicity	.94	42, 2625	0.96

*$p < .05$. **$p < .01$. ***$p < .001$.

to conclude that sleep in general significantly varies across these main effects and the one interaction. Univariate testing of the individual sleep variables then reveals which measures changed with which factor.

The results for the main and interaction effects associated with ethnicity are presented in chapter 6. For now, we should bear in mind that univariate results for the main effects of ethnicity found significant differences between AA and CA for SOL, SE, and NAP. Also, the age × ethnicity interaction was significant for TST and NAP. We now turn to the univariate results to explore in detail the sleep measures for the main effects of age and gender.

Main Effects of Age

To clarify our age reference system, we often refer to a decade by its lower boundary as done on the abscissa of the figures. For example, decade 30 refers to participants in the 30–39 age range and decade 70 refers to individuals in the 70–79 age range.

We begin with presenting the relevant raw data for the main effect of Age. Table 4.3 presents means (and SDs) for sleep measures by age decade. These data were extracted from the Whole Sample, Total column of Appendix Tables A4.1 to A4.7. Table 4.3 is intended as an archive, but includes too great an amount of information to convey a clear picture of sleep and aging by itself. The subsequent discussion of sleep changes across the life span and the accompanying figures rely on the data from Table 4.3, and attempt to isolate the differences in particular measures observed across the life span.

Table 4.4 reveals that most of the sleep measures (NWAK, WASO, TST, SQR, and NAP) exhibited significant change across the life span. Only two of the age measures, SOL and SE, did not register significant change between age groups.

We now present line plots to more clearly illuminate the significant univariate results for the main effects of age. These are accompanied by trend analyses that focus our attention on critical changes across decades.

SOL. This variable fluctuated within the 17.2 min to 20.5 min range (Table 4.3 and Fig. 4.1). The nonsignificant peak was reached in decade 80, and the nonsignificant low occurred in decade 60. Given that SOL age change was nonsignificant, it is fair to consider an overall SOL value in the broad normal sample. This conclusion is supported by the absence of a significant univariate effect for SOL within the age × ethnicity interaction and a nonsignificant univariate gender effect for this

TABLE 4.3

Broad Normal Sample: Mean (SD) for Sleep Measures by Age

Variable	Decade 20–29 (n = 91)		Decade 30–39 (n = 97)		Decade 40–49 (n = 79)		Decade 50–59 (n = 92)		Decade 60–69 (n = 89)		Decade 70–79 (n = 80)		Decade 80–89+ (n = 65)	
	M	SD	M	SD	M	SD	M	SD	M	SD	M	SD	M	SD
SOL	19.2	12.5	17.9	11.8	18.8	15.0	17.6	14.3	17.2	12.3	20.1	16.3	20.5	11.1
NWAK	1.1	1.0	1.2	0.8	1.2	0.9	1.3	1.0	1.5	1.0	1.6	0.9	1.8	1.1
WASO	15.2	18.3	15.8	20.0	16.6	18.4	13.0	12.2	22.6	23.2	21.7	19.2	26.0	23.8
TST	439.3	66.7	413.6	53.5	406.9	51.9	415.1	58.9	428.7	61.1	428.7	63.6	461.8	71.0
SE	89.1	6.0	88.6	7.0	88.2	9.0	89.6	5.9	88.0	7.5	87.8	6.0	87.0	7.2
SQR	3.4	0.5	3.5	0.7	3.5	0.6	3.6	0.6	3.7	0.7	3.6	0.7	3.7	0.7
NAP	14.2	19.9	15.4	19.1	11.3	15.1	12.5	18.3	18.3	25.7	19.3	24.2	24.2	21.2

TABLE 4.4
Broad Normal Sample: ANOVA Results for Sleep Measures by Age

Variable	F
SOL	0.75
NWAK	4.00**
WASO	3.05**
TST	9.26***
SE	1.29
SQR	2.64*
NAP	4.01**

Note. All dfs are 6, 565. *$p < .05$. **$p < .01$. ***$p < .001$.

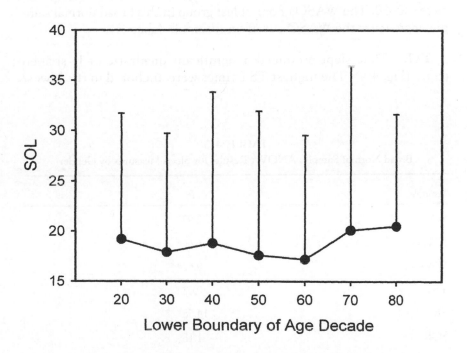

FIG. 4.1.   Mean (and SD bar) sleep onset latency (minutes) by decade in the broad normal sample. There were no significant differences between age groups.

variable (Table 4.5). Among the 593 participants in this sample, we observed SOL to be 18.6 min, $SD = 13.4$. However, this conclusion is tempered somewhat by a main effect for ethnicity for SOL, and we return to these data in chapter 6.

NWAK. Awakenings produced a linear trend, meaning the positive slope of the linear representation of the increment in NWAK over the life span was statistically significant (Fig. 4.2). Awakenings went from a low of 1.1 per night in decade 20 to nearly doubling with a high of 1.8 per night in decade 80. Except for the leveling off in decades 30 and 40, the increase in NWAK from one decade to the next was gradual and steady, never dramatic.

WASO. Time awake also produced a significant linear trend (Fig. 4.3), although its path along the life span was not so regular as was with NWAK. The low WASO was 13.0 min in decade 50 and the high was 26.0 min in decade 80. WASO during decades 60–80 doubled that of decades 20–50. The WASO of our oldest group in this broad normal sample approaches the WASO cutoff for insomnia (chap. 5).

TST. Time slept produced a significant quadratic or U-shaped trend (Fig. 4.4). The highest TST times were anchored in the lowest

TABLE 4.5
Broad Normal Sample: ANOVA Results for Sleep Measures by Gender

Variable	F
SOL	2.92
NWAK	6.66*
WASO	9.62**
TST	0.02
SE	14.58***
SQR	1.18
NAP	0.10

Note. All dfs are 1, 565. *$p < .05$. **$p < .01$. ***$p < .001$.

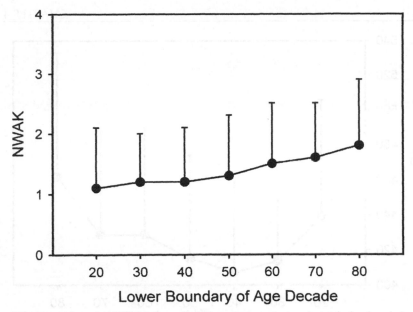

FIG. 4.2. Mean (and *SD* bar) number of awakenings during the night by decade in the broad normal sample. There was a significant linear trend for increasing number of awakenings with advancing age.

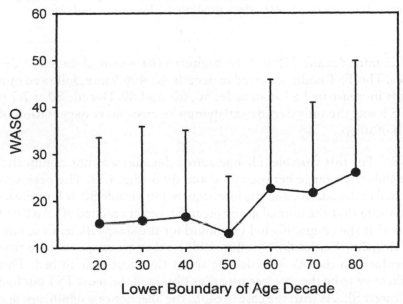

FIG. 4.3. Mean (and *SD* bar) wake time after sleep onset (minutes) by decade in the broad normal sample. There was a significant linear trend for increasing wake time after sleep onset with advancing age.

83

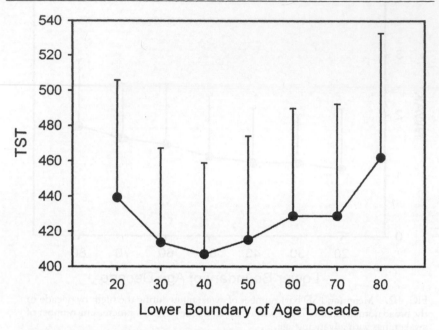

FIG. 4.4.   Mean (and SD bar) total sleep time (minutes) by decade in the broad normal sample. There was a significant quadratic trend for total sleep time across the life span.

(439.3 min, decade 20) and the highest (461.8 min, decade 80) de-cades. The TST nadir occurred in decade 40, 406.9 min, followed by a steady increase in TST in decades 50, 60, and 80. Decade 80 at 7.7 h of TST was the only decade satisfying the customary expectation of 7.5 h of sleep.

SE.   For this variable, change across decades was not significant. SE exhibited a range between 87.0 and 89.6 (Fig. 4.5). The peak was reached in decade 50, and the low occurred in decade 80. It is interest-ing to note that the normal group mean SE never reached 90. An SE of 90 to 95 is the commonly held standard for the sleep efficiency of nor-mal sleepers (Kupfer & Reynolds, 1983). Also, we may conclude that individuals in the 80–89+ decade spent the most time in bed. This would have to be the case because they obtained the most TST but had the lowest SE. As with the case of SOL, the absence of a significant age × ethnicity interaction for SE permits us to consider an aggregate value for this measure, but significant main effects for both gender (Ta-ble 4.5) and ethnicity for SE cause us to consider this aggregate cau-

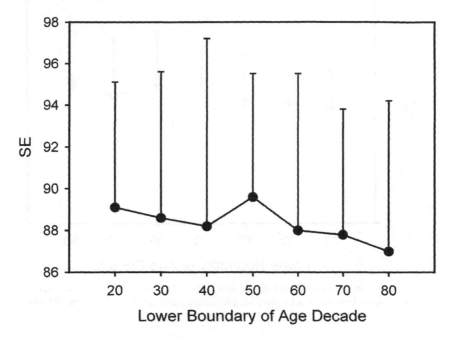

FIG. 4.5.   Mean (and *SD* bar) sleep efficiency percent (TST/TIB × 100) by decade in the broad normal sample. There were no significant differences between age groups.

tiously. Among the 593 participants in the broad normal sample, SE averaged 88.4, $SD = 7.0$.

SQR.   Rated quality of sleep produced a significant linear trend, indicating perceived sleep quality gradually rises over the life span within the fair (score of 3) to good (score of 4) range (Fig. 4.6). SQR rose from a low of 3.4 (high fair rating) in decade 20 to a high of 3.7 (low good rating) in decade 80. Even though this gradual rise in SQR across the life span is statistically significant, the magnitude of change is not great. However, it is noteworthy that rated quality of sleep improves over the life span, rather than the opposite.

NAP.   Daytime sleeping produced a significant quadratic trend, albeit a messy U-shape (Fig. 4.7). In general, napping is moderately high in the young adult years (decades 20 and 30), dips during the middle years (decades 40 and 50), and peaks in the later years (decades 60–80). The three highest napping decades occurred in the later years, decades 60,

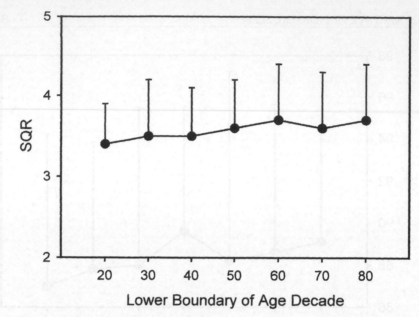

FIG. 4.6.   Mean (and *SD* bar) sleep quality rating (from 1 = *very poor* to 5 = excellent) by decade in the broad normal sample. There was a significant linear trend for increasing sleep quality rating with advancing age.

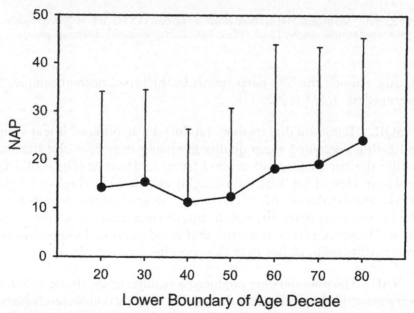

FIG. 4.7.   Mean (and *SD* bar) time spent napping (minutes) by decade in the broad normal sample. There was a significant quadratic trend for time spent napping across the life span.

70, and 80. The peak of 24.2 min occurred in decade 80. A minor peak occurred in decade 30, 15.4 min. The napping nadir occurred in decade 40, 11.3 min. Decade 80 also exhibited the peak TST (Table 4.3). Combining NAP and TST, 80–89 + was the only decade in which sleep during a 24-h period exceeded (by about 5 min) 8 h.

Summary.   Five of seven sleep measures registered significant change across the life span—NWAK, WASO, TST, SQR, and NAP—and two measures did not significantly change across age groups: SOL and SE. Of the five measures that changed, three reflected worse sleep with advancing age: NWAK, WASO, and NAPS. These changes were not always regular (linear) from decade to decade, and this conclusion also assumes that increasing nap time is a negative indicator reflecting an inadequate nighttime sleep experience and a fragmented sleep pattern.

Two measures improved, SQR and TST. The changes with SQR were very regular across decades, but TST changes were nonlinear, although finally peaking in old age.

Review of Fig. 4.1 to 4.7 reveals a clear old age effect in three variables: WASO, TST, and NAPS. For these measures, aging *bumps* occurred at decade 60, although not always negative. It is equally revealing that no sharp old age change occurred with the remaining four sleep variables.

Main Effects of Gender

Table 4.5 presents the univariate results for gender. Differences between men and women were statistically significant for three measures, NWAK, WASO, and SE.

Table 4.6 presents the means (and *SDs*) for the main effects of gender. We now see that for all three significant variables, women slept worse: NWAK men, $M = 1.3$, women, $M = 1.4$; WASO men, $M = 16.4$, women, $M = 20.2$; SE men, $M = 89.4$, women, $M = 87.4$. However, the magnitude of these differences is small. Factoring in the nonsignificant differences in the remaining four measures, we conclude that the difference in sleep between men and women is not great in the broad normal sample.

NARROW NORMAL SAMPLE: SLEEP
BY AGE, GENDER, AND ETHNICITY

As with the broad normal sample, we began with a three-factor MANOVA, 7 age decades × 2 gender × 2 ethnicity for seven sleep measures, SOL, NWAK, WASO, TST, SE, SQR, and NAP. The results of this analysis are summarized in Table 4.7.

TABLE 4.6
Broad Normal Sample: Mean and SD for Sleep Measures by Gender

Variable	Men		Women	
	M	SD	M	SD
SOL	17.1	11.8	20.2	14.7
NWAK*	1.3	1.0	1.4	0.9
WASO**	16.4	19.5	20.2	20.0
TST	425.6	64.0	427.3	61.4
SE***	89.4	6.5	87.4	7.3
SQR	3.6	0.6	3.5	0.6
NAP	16.2	21.2	16.0	20.8

*$p < .05$. **$p < .01$. ***$p < .001$.

TABLE 4.7
Narrow Normal Sample: MANOVA Results for Sleep Measures by Age, Gender, and Ethnicity

Factor	Wilks' Λ	df	F Equivalent
Age	.69	42, 1682	3.32***
Gender	.96	7, 358	2.44*
Ethnicity	.91	7, 358	5.45***
Age × gender	.85	42, 1682	1.46*
Age × ethnicity	.88	42, 1682	1.20
Gender × ethnicity	.97	7, 358	1.65
Age × gender × ethnicity	.87	42, 1682	1.29

*$p < .05$. ***$p < .001$.

We again found significant main effects for our three factors, age, gender, and ethnicity. We may then conclude that sleep in general differs between groups in each of these factors. We found a different significant interaction, age × gender, than was found with the broad normal sample.

Here too, the results for the main effects associated with ethnicity are presented in chapter 6. For now, we should bear in mind that univariate results for the main effects of ethnicity found significant differences between AA and CA for the same variables as the broad normal sample, SOL, SE, and NAP. We now turn to the univariate results to explore in detail the sleep measures for the main effects of age and gender, and the interaction of these two factors.

Main Effects of Age

Table 4.8 presents means (and SDs) for sleep measures by age decade in the narrow normal sample. These data were extracted from the Whole Sample, Total column of Appendix Tables A4.8 to A4.14. The subsequent discussion of sleep changes across the life span and the accompanying figures rely on the data from Table 4.8.

Significant univariate sleep effects across age decades were obtained with five measures: NWAK, WASO, TST, SQR, and NAP (Table 4.9). SOL and SE did not exhibit significant change across the life span. This pattern of significance exactly matches that obtained for the main effects of age in the broad normal sample.

We now proceed with the results of trend analysis and presentation of age effects in figures. Three of these variables showed a significant age × gender interaction: NWAK, WASO, and NAP. Analyses and figures for these three are reserved for the interaction section that follows.

SOL. Time to fall asleep ranged from 12.8 to 15.9 min and these differences were nonsignificant (Table 4.8 and Fig. 4.8). SOL peaked early, decade 20, and reached its nadir in decade 60. SOL ethnic differences are explored in chapter 6. Given nonsignificant age and gender effects for SOL, we consider a summary value. For this sample of 392 pristine sleepers, SOL averaged 14.3 min (SD = 8.7).

TST. This variable exhibited a significant quadratic trend (Fig. 4.9), declining from young adult to middle age, and then rising again in the later years. Peaks were reached in the lowest (decade 20, M = 445.6 min, SD = 48.7) and highest (decade 80, M = 475.0 min, SD = 77.0) age

TABLE 4.8
Narrow Normal Sample: Mean (SD) for Sleep Measures by Age

Variable	Decade 20–29 (n = 68)		Decade 30–39 n = 64		Decade 40–49 (n = 59)		Decade 50–59 (n = 60)		Decade 60–69 (n = 58)		Decade 70–79 (n = 47)		Decade 80–89+ (n = 36)	
	M	SD	M	SD	M	SD	M	SD	M	SD	M	SD	M	SD
SOL	15.9	5.9	13.9	7.5	13.6	7.6	13.3	8.0	12.8	6.3	15.5	15.3	15.4	8.7
NWAK	0.9	0.8	1.0	0.7	1.1	0.8	1.1	1.0	1.3	0.9	1.5	0.9	1.4	1.0
WASO	9.3	7.9	9.8	7.8	11.4	10.0	8.9	7.6	11.6	9.7	13.4	10.2	13.6	10.1
TST	445.6	48.7	424.2	46.5	414.7	46.2	414.1	63.2	438.6	54.1	436.6	65.2	475.0	77.0
SE	91.5	3.4	91.3	4.0	91.2	4.9	91.3	4.6	91.4	4.8	90.7	4.1	91.1	3.8
SQR	3.5	0.5	3.7	0.6	3.6	0.6	3.8	0.5	3.9	0.6	3.6	0.7	4.0	0.5
NAP	12.3	19.1	11.5	13.1	8.3	11.4	12.5	21.1	13.3	15.6	18.4	18.8	20.5	18.6

TABLE 4.9
Narrow Normal Sample: ANOVA Results for Sleep Measures by Age

Variable	F
SOL	0.80
NWAK	3.75**
WASO	3.35**
TST	6.83***
SE	0.38
SQR	2.78*
NAP	4.06**

Note. All *dfs* are 6, 364. *p < .05. **p < .01. ***p < .001.

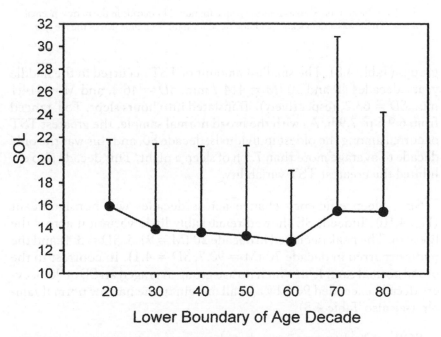

FIG. 4.8.   Mean (and *SD* bar) sleep onset latency (minutes) by decade in the narrow normal sample. There were no significant differences between age groups.

91

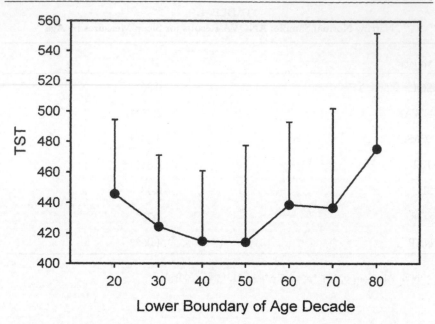

FIG. 4.9.   Mean (and *SD* bar) total sleep time (minutes) by decade in the narrow normal sample. There was a significant quadratic trend for total sleep time across the life span.

groups (Table 4.8). The smallest amount of TST occurred in the middle years, decades 40 and 50 ($M = 414.7$ min, $SD = 46.2$, and $M = 414.1$ min, $SD = 63.2$, respectively). Translated into hours slept, TST ranged from 6.9 h to 7.9 h. As with the broad normal sample, the greatest TST occurred among the oldest individuals, decade 80, and this was the only decade to average more than 7.5 h of sleep a night. This decade also exhibited the greatest TST variability.

SE.   Sleep efficiency change across decades was nonsignificant (Fig. 4.10). Indeed, SE showed remarkably little variation across the lifespan. The peak occurred in decade 20 ($M = 91.5$, $SD = 3.4$) and the nadir occurred in decade 70 ($M = 90.7$, $SD = 4.1$). In contrast to the broad normal sample in which no age group averaged an SE of 90%, every decade exceeded 90% by a small margin in the narrow normal sample (see also Table 4.8).

SQR.   Quality ratings produced an uncommon significant quintic pattern (Fig. 4.11). Such a pattern is characterized by four *turns*, occurring at decade 30, 40, 60, and 70. The quintic pattern traced a rise

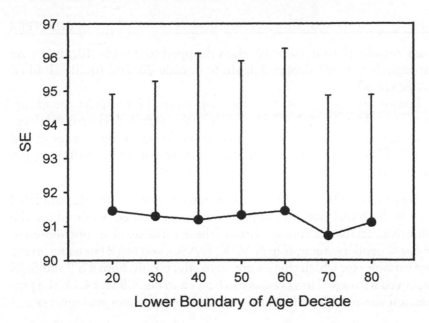

FIG. 4.10.   Mean (and *SD* bar) sleep efficiency percent (TST/TIB × 100) by decade in the narrow normal sample. There were no significant differences between age groups.

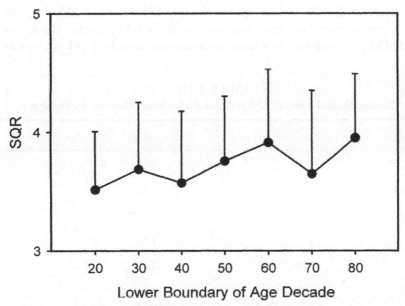

FIG. 4.11.   Mean (and *SD* bar) sleep quality rating (from 1 = *very poor* to 5 = excellent) by decade in the narrow normal sample. There was a significant quintic trend for sleep quality rating across the life span.

from decade 20 to decade 30, then dropped to decade 40, then rose through decade 60, dropped again to decade 70, and finally climbed to decade 80.

Lowest rated sleep satisfaction occurred in the youngest age group, decade 20 ($M = 3.5, SD = 0.5$), and this value signaled fair to good sleep. The highest rated sleep occurred in the oldest age group, decade 80 ($M = 4.0, SD = 0.5$). Among all decades in the broad and narrow samples, this was the only one to average a *good* rating.

Summary. The age pattern in the narrow normal sample paralleled that of the broad normal sample. Significant change occurred for the same five variables, although three of these variables also contributed to an age × gender interaction: NWAK, WASO, and NAP. Focusing on the two variables for which there were main effects only, both TST and SQR improved with age. However, as can be seen in Fig. 4.9 and 4.11, the progression was not linear but rather marked by advances and reverses.

Main Effects of Gender

Table 4.10 presents the univariate results derived from the main effects of gender. Of the seven sleep measures, only NWAK and WASO significantly distinguished the men and women. Table 4.11 presents the means (and SDs) for gender within the narrow normal sample. For both signifi-

TABLE 4.10
Narrow Normal Sample: ANOVA Results for Sleep Measures by Gender

Variable	F
SOL	0.03
NWAK	6.31*
WASO	13.25***
TST	1.53
SE	3.86
SQR	0.28
NAP	0.07

Note. All *dfs* are 1, 364. *$p < .05$. ***$p < .001$.

TABLE 4.11
Narrow Normal Sample: Mean and SD for Sleep Measures by Gender

	Men		Women	
Variable	M	SD	M	SD
SOL	14.0	8.0	14.6	9.4
NWAK*	1.1	0.9	1.2	0.9
WASO***	10.1	8.4	11.8	9.7
TST	429.4	58.7	437.7	58.6
SE	91.5	4.2	90.9	4.3
SQR	3.7	0.6	3.7	0.6
NAP	14.4	19.0	11.9	14.8

*$p < .05$. ***$p < .001$.

cant variables, women slept worse by a small magnitude. NWAK and WASO also contributed to the significant age × gender interaction, and these data are later discussed further.

Age × Gender Interaction

Significant interaction was found for three measures: NWAK, WASO, and NAP (Table 4.12). Table 4.13 presents the data on which the analysis of simple effects of this interaction are based. These data were extracted from the Whole Sample, Men and Women columns of Appendix Tables A4.8 to A4.14.

We proceed with reporting the analysis of simple effects. Interpretation of these data are aided by bar graphs.

NWAK. For the simple effects of age, we found a significant linear trend for both men and women. Referring to Table 4.13 and Fig. 4.12, this linear trend means NWAK gradually rises in both groups across the life span, despite plateaus (women in decades 20–60) and abrupt peaks (men in decade 60). For men, low NWAK occurs in decade 20 and peaks in decade 60. For women, NWAK is stable in the range of 1 to 1.2 number of awakenings through decade 60 and then jumps up to 1.6 in

TABLE 4.12

Narrow Normal Sample: ANOVA Results for Sleep Measures
by the Age × Gender Interaction

Variable	F
SOL	0.50
NWAK	3.17**
WASO	2.67*
TST	0.26
SE	1.04
SQR	0.82
NAP	2.48*

Note. All *dfs* are 6, 364. *$p < .05$. **$p < .01$.

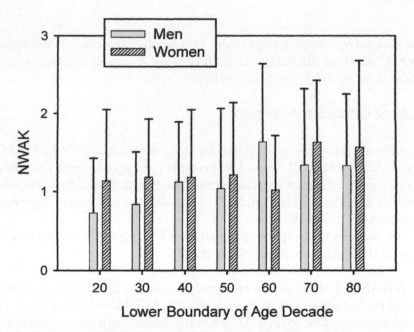

FIG. 4.12. Mean (and *SD* bar) number of awakenings during the night by gender and decade in the narrow normal sample. There was a significant linear trend for increasing number of awakenings with advancing age among both men and women. Significant gender differences occurred in decades 20 and 60.

TABLE 4.13

Narrow Normal Sample: Mean (SD) for Sleep Measures Showing an Age × Gender Interaction

Variable	Decade 20–29		Decade 30–39		Decade 40–49		Decade 50–59		Decade 60–69		Decade 70–79		Decade 80–89+	
	M	SD	M	SD	M	SD	M	SD	M	SD	M	SD	M	SD
NWAK														
Men	0.7	0.7	0.8	0.7	1.1	0.8	1.0	1.0	1.6	1.0	1.3	1.0	1.3	0.9
Women	1.1	0.9	1.2	0.7	1.2	0.9	1.2	0.9	1.0	0.7	1.6	0.8	1.6	1.1
WASO														
Men	7.0	5.5	8.8	8.4	11.7	10.8	8.8	7.8	11.7	8.4	10.3	6.5	12.9	9.8
Women	11.7	9.4	10.7	7.1	10.9	9.0	8.9	7.6	11.6	11.0	17.3	12.6	15.0	11.0
NAP														
Men	11.7	20.6	8.8	12.5	10.2	13.1	14.3	26.0	16.9	17.0	23.9	20.5	17.8	17.4
Women	12.8	17.7	14.0	13.4	5.5	7.7	10.5	13.8	9.5	13.1	11.6	14.1	26.0	20.6

the last two decades. For the simple effects of gender, Fig. 4.12 shows that NWAK is close between the two groups in most decades. Significant differences were found in decades 20 (women significantly higher) and 60 (men significantly higher). Women had a higher NWAK in every decade but 60.

WASO.   For the simple effects of age, as with NWAK, we found a significant linear trend for both men and women. Referring to Table 4.13 and Fig. 4.13, although the increase is not perfectly regular, WASO gradually rises in both groups across the life span. For men, low WASO occurs in decade 20 and peaks in decade 80. For women, WASO is stable in the range of 8.9 to 11.7 min through decade 60 and then jumps up to 17 and 15 min in the last two decades. For the simple effects of gender, Fig. 4.13 shows that WASO is close between the two groups in most decades. Sig-

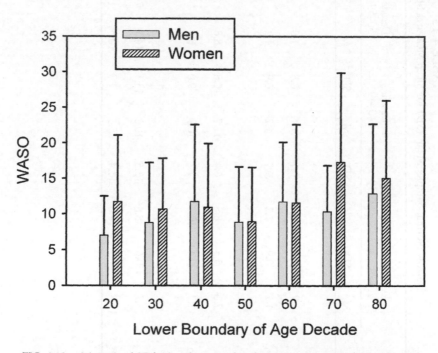

FIG. 4.13.   Mean (and *SD* bar) wake time after sleep onset (minutes) by gender and decade in the narrow normal sample. There was a significant linear trend for increasing wake time after sleep onset with advancing age among both men and women. Significant gender differences occurred in decades 20 and 70.

nificant differences were found in decades 20 and 70, and in both cases women had higher WASO. Women had a higher WASO, often by a small margin, in five of seven decades.

NAP. For the simple effects of age, we found a significant linear trend for men and a quadratic trend for women. Referring to Table 4.13 and Fig. 4.14, NAP gradually rises in men across the life span, again by an irregular pattern. For men, low NAP occurs in decade 30 (8.8 min) and peaks in decade 70 (23.9 min). For women, the trend is captured by a U-shaped pattern. There are napping peaks in the low end in decades 20 and 30; NAP then dips and is low and steady in decades 40 to 70 (range 5.5 to 11.6 min), and finally jumps up to 26 min in decade 80. For the simple effects of gender, a significant difference was found in decade 70 only (men nap more than women).

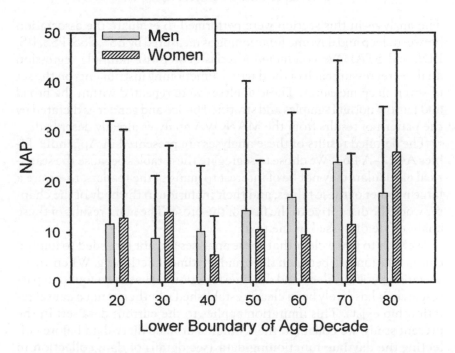

FIG. 4.14.   Mean (and SD bar) time spent napping (minutes) by gender and decade in the narrow normal sample. There was a significant linear trend for increasing time spent napping with advancing age among men and a significant quadratic trend for time spent napping across the life span for women. Significant gender differences occurred in decade 70.

Summary. The age × gender interaction affected three sleep variables in the narrow normal sample. Some overriding themes can be extracted from these data.

NWAK and WASO exhibited generally similar patterns. Both these aspects of sleep became more problematic with advancing age, and differences between men and women were not great, although women's sleep on these two measures tended to be worse.

The NAP pattern was more distinctive. Although men and women tended to increase napping in the later years, men increased their napping by regular increments across the life span, whereas women's napping decreased in the middle years before increasing in the later years. Differences in NAP between men and woman varied across the life span, but here greater NAP tended to occur among men.

ASSOCIATION BETWEEN SLEEP
AND DAYTIME FUNCTIONING

The analyses in this section were performed to evaluate the association between sleep and daytime functioning as measured by ESS, SSS, FSS, IIS, BDI, and STAI. We conducted a series of stepwise multiple regression analyses regressing each of the daytime functioning instruments on the set of seven sleep measures. These analyses were repeated within the broad and narrow normal samples and stratified by age and gender as dictated by the pattern of results from the MANOVA analyses already described.

The detailed results of these analyses are presented in Appendix Tables A4.22–A4.67. We chose to segregate these tables because the statistical particulars may not be of interest to many of the readers, there are a large number of these tables, and their inclusion in the body of the chapter would be disruptive to the flow of the prose. The main results of these analyses are discussed in the text.

We wish to make clear that these analyses are not intended to imply a causal relationship between sleep and daytime functioning. When an association between sleep and daytime functioning has been found in past research, it has rarely been clearly established whether or not a causal relationship exists. This limitation applies to the current data set. In the present study, we collected the 14 nights of sleep diary data before collecting the daytime functioning data (see details of data collection in chap. 3). This temporal sequence persuaded us to view sleep as a predictor of daytime functioning. Nevertheless, when we find associations in the following analyses, the question of causal inference remains indeterminate. Further, were causality present, the current methodology could not determine if daytime functioning altered sleep or sleep altered daytime functioning.

Broad Normal Sample

Analyses relating to ethnicity are be reserved for chapter 6. There remains in the broad normal sample main effects for age and gender. To accommodate these results in the regression analyses, we dichotomized age as young (decades 20, 30, 40, and 50) and old (decades 60, 70, and 80). Most of the sleep measures changed with age, and these cutoffs fit our data reasonably well and also fit common sleep research practice in other labs in exploring age affects. Therefore, we conduct four sets of regression analyses: the young group, the old group, men, and women. Only significant results are reported.

Sleep and Daytime Functioning in the Young Group.   Four sleep variables accounted for 11% of the variance in ESS (Table A4.22). As would be expected, poorer SQR, longer NAP, and increased NWAK were associated with greater daytime sleepiness as measured by the ESS. Shorter SOL was associated with higher ESS scores, and this is a little bit more difficult to interpret. Plausibly, higher levels of daytime sleepiness promote shorter sleep onset at bedtime. NWAK was weighted less heavily (contributed less explained variance) than the other sleep variables.

Two sleep variable accounted for 8% of the variance in SSS (Table A4.23). Predictably, poorer SQR and longer NAP were associated with greater daytime sleepiness as measured by the SSS, and SQR was weighted more heavily than NAP.

One sleep variable accounted for 6% of the variance in FSS (Table A4.24). Poorer SQR was associated with greater daytime fatigue as measured by the FSS.

Greater negative impact of insomnia as measured by the IIS was associated with poorer SQR, more TST, and more NAP (Table A4.25). We cannot explain why more TST is related to higher IIS scores. These three sleep measures accounted for 17% of the variance in IIS, with SQR being the dominant factor.

SQR was again the main correlate of daytime functioning as measured by the BDI, accounting for 10% of variability (Table A4.26). WASO provided another 2% of explained variability. In both cases, poorer sleep measure scores were associated with a higher depression rating.

Only SQR was associated with STAI, but the strength of the relationship was substantial (Table A4.27). Lower SQR was related to higher STAI (14% explained variability).

Summary. Table 4.14 presents a summary of findings for the relationship between sleep and daytime functioning among young adults in the broad normal sample. Positive and negative signs were inserted in the matrix of sleep by daytime measures to indicate the presence and direction of significant associations. For example, the negative signs for SQR mean that lower SQR scores (poorer sleep quality) were associated with higher scores on the daytime functioning measures, which in all cases meant poorer daytime functioning.

In total, we found 13 significant relationships, and more than half of these involved SQR. Not only was SQR most frequently related to daytime functioning, but it consistently accounted for greater explained variance than the other sleep measures.

Participants mainly perceived a relationship between two sleep variables, SQR and to a lesser degree NAP, and daytime functioning. SE did not appear at all, and four other measures, SOL, NWAK, WASO, and

TABLE 4.14
Summary of Regression Analyses: Broad Normal Sample, Young Adults

Sleep Measures	Measures of Daytime Functioning					
	ESS	SSS	FSS	IIS	BDI	STAI
SOL	−					
NWAK	+					
WASO					+	
TST				+		
SE						
SQR	−	−	−	−	−	−
NAP	+	+		+		

Note. Signs indicate the presence and direction of the relationship between the sleep and daytime functioning measures.

TST, appeared only once. Two findings appeared that were inconsistent with our expectations. SOL and ESS were negatively correlated, and TST and IIS were positively correlated.

Sleep and Daytime Functioning in the Old Group. The daytime sleepiness variables, ESS and SSS, showed a similar pattern (Tables A4.28 and A4.29). NAP was the only predictor significantly related to these measures, accounting for 12% and 14% explained variance respectively. In both cases, increased napping was associated with higher sleepiness scores among older adults.

Increased NAP (6% variance explained), increased TST (2%), and decreased SE (4%) predicted FSS (Table A4.30). The NAP and SE associations are plausible, but why more TST predicts greater fatigue is not readily apparent.

Four variables accounted for 11% of the variance in IIS (Table A4.31). Greater NAP, SOL, and TST and lower SQR were associated with greater insomnia impact. NAP and SOL were weighted more heavily than the other two. Here again, the positive correlation with TST is somewhat puzzling.

Lower SQR was the main predictor of both BDI and STAI (Tables A4.32 and A4.33). More NAP and more TST also predicted BDI, but these were not weighted as heavily as SQR. An unexpected but fairly consistent pattern of more sleep time associated with impaired daytime functioning has emerged. More NAP was the second variable associated with STAI, although its contribution to explained variance was about a fourth that of SQR.

Summary. Fourteen significant relationships were found between sleep and daytime functioning in this group, and half involved NAP (Table 4.15). Not only did old adults perceive a relationship between NAP and every daytime variable, but the weight of the NAP contribution was often the strongest of the sleep variables. SQR was relevant for three daytime variables. We continue to see what will be a very consistent finding: Increased TST predicts diminished daytime functioning.

Sleep and Daytime Functioning in Men. Results for the two sleepiness measures, ESS (10% variance explained) and SSS (7% variance explained), were similar (Tables A4.34 and A4.35). More NAP and lower SQR were associated with increased daytime sleepiness. For both ESS and SSS, NAP was weighted more heavily than SQR.

TABLE 4.15
Summary of Regression Analyses: Broad Normal Sample, Old Adults

	Measures of Daytime Functioning					
Sleep Measures	ESS	SSS	FSS	IIS	BDI	STAI
SOL				+		
NWAK						
WASO						
TST			+	+	+	
SE			−			
SQR			−		−	−
NAP	+	+	+	+	+	+

Note. Signs indicate the presence and direction of the relationship between the sleep and daytime functioning measures.

Results for fatigue (FSS, 9% variance explained) and general insomnia impact (IIS, 8% variance explained) were also similar (Tables A4.36 and A4.37). Low SQR and high NAP and TST predicted both. SQR was the strongest predictor for both measures, but the sequence of NAP and TST varied. Increased TST associated with diminished daytime functioning appears counterintuitive.

Four variables accounted for 18% of the variability in BDI (Table A4.38). Low SQR (8% variance explained), high NAP (7%), high TST (2%), and low SE (1%) were associated with elevated depression. All of these relationships, except for TST, are as expected.

There occurred only one significant predictor of STAI (Table A4.39). Low SQR (11% variance explained) related to greater anxiety.

Summary. We found 15 significant relationships in this group, and this was almost entirely based in SQR and NAP (Table 4.16). Men in the broad normal sample perceived a relationship between NAP and SQR with every daytime variable except NAP with STAI. Overall, NAP and SQR were weighted about equally. Three variables, SOL, NWAK, and WASO, were unrelated to any measure of daytime functioning. In-

TABLE 4.16
Summary of Regression Analyses: Broad Normal Sample, Men

	Measures of Daytime Functioning					
Sleep Measures	ESS	SSS	FSS	IIS	BDI	STAI
SOL						
NWAK						
WASO						
TST			+	+	+	
SE					−	
SQR	−	−	−	−	−	−
NAP	+	+	+	+	+	

Note. Signs indicate the presence and direction of the relationship between the sleep and daytime functioning measures.

creased TST predicted diminished daytime functioning for three variables, FSS, IIS, and BDI.

Sleep and Daytime Functioning in Women. NAP (7% explained variance) and SOL (2%) were associated with ESS (Table A4.40). More NAP and, surprisingly, shorter SOL predicted increased daytime sleepiness in women.

Two sleep variables also related to SSS (Table A4.41). Higher NAP (10% explained variance) and lower SQR (2%) were associated with SSS.

Three variables predicted 5% of the variability in FSS (Table A4.42). Low SQR (weighted most heavily), high TST, and low SE were associated with fatigue. The TST finding is again surprising, although it accounted for only 1% of variance.

Four sleep variables accounted for 20% of the variance in IIS (Table A4.43). Low SQR and NWAK and high NAP and TST predicted greater IIS impairment. The NWAK and the TST findings are counterintuitive. SQR supplied the bulk of the explained variance (14%) for this variable.

SQR was the sole predictor of BDI and STAI (Tables A4.44 and A4.45). Low SQR accounted for 10% and 16% of variance, respectively, for these two measures.

Summary. For women in the broad normal sample, SQR and NAP continue to be the strongest predictors of daytime functioning among the 13 significant relationships that emerged (Table 4.17). Paradoxical findings occurred with TST and NWAK.

Narrow Normal Sample

Because there was an age × gender interaction in the narrow normal sample, the analytic strategy had to be modified from that used with the broad normal sample. We again use the two age groups as defined for the broad normal sample, young (decades 20, 30, 40, and 50) and old (decades 60, 70, and 80). We then analyze gender within age groups, creating four sets of analyses: young men, young women, old men, and old women.

Sleep and Daytime Functioning in the Young Men Group. SQR was the only sleep variable related to the first three daytime function measures: ESS, SSS, and FSS (Tables A4.46, A4.47,and A4.48). In all cases, poorer sleep ratings were associated with diminished daytime functioning, with explained variance occurring within the 5% to 8% range.

TABLE 4.17
Summary of Regression Analyses: Broad Normal Sample, Women

| Sleep Measures | Measures of Daytime Functioning | | | | | |
	ESS	SSS	FSS	IIS	BDI	STAI
SOL	−					
NWAK				−		
WASO						
TST			+	+		
SE			−			
SQR		−	−	−	−	−
NAP	+	+		+		

Note. Signs indicate the presence and direction of the relationship between the sleep and daytime functioning measures.

Lower SQR (10% explained variance), higher TST (4%),and higher NAP (3%) were related to higher IIS scores (Table A4.49). The consistent but surprising finding that more sleep is associated with poorer daytime functioning was replicated here.

Greater WASO was associated with higher BDI scores (Table A4.50). WASO accounted for 7% of the variability in BDI.

Lower SQR was associated with higher STAI scores (Table A4.51). SQR accounted for 13% of the variability in STAI.

Summary. Eight significant relationships were found (Table 4.18). For young men in the narrow normal sample, SQR was the sole strong predictor of daytime functioning. Paradoxical findings occurred with TST and NWAK.

Sleep and Daytime Functioning in the Young Women Group. NAP was the sole sleep measure related to ESS (7% explained variance) and SSS (11% explained variance) (Tables A4.52 and A4.53). In both cases, increased napping was associated with higher scores on these two measures of sleepiness.

TABLE 4.18
Summary of Regression Analyses: Narrow Normal Sample, Young Men

| Sleep Measures | Measures of Daytime Functioning | | | | | |
	ESS	SSS	FSS	IIS	BDI	STAI
SOL						
NWAK						
WASO					+	
TST				+		
SE						
SQR	−	−	−	−		−
NAP				+		

Note. Signs indicate the presence and direction of the relationship between the sleep and daytime functioning measures.

SQR was the sole sleep variable related to the remaining four measures in the young women subset: FSS, IIS, BDI, and STAI (Tables A4.54, A4.55, A4.56, and A4.57). In all cases, lower SQR was associated with diminished daytime functioning. Explained variance ranged from 6% to 10% for FSS, IIS, and BDI. It jumped up to 18% for STAI.

Summary.   For young women in the narrow normal sample, no more than one sleep variable was associated with any aspect of daytime functioning (Table 4.19). SQR predominated in predicting daytime functioning. NAP was the sole sleep measure associated with measures of daytime sleepiness. No other sleep variable predicted any of our daytime measures.

Sleep and Daytime Functioning in the Old Men Group.   NAP predicted 16% of the variance in ESS (Table A4.58). Increased NAP was associated with increased ESS.

WASO predicted 5% of the variance in SSS (Table A4.59). Increased WASO was associated with increased SSS.

NAP predicted 10% of the variance in FSS (Table A4.60). Increased NAP was associated with increased FSS.

TABLE 4.19
Summary of Regression Analyses: Narrow Normal Sample, Young Women

Sleep Measures	ESS	SSS	FSS	IIS	BDI	STAI
			Measures of Daytime Functioning			
SOL						
NWAK						
WASO						
TST						
SE						
SQR			−	−	−	−
NAP	+	+				

Note. Signs indicate the presence and direction of the relationship between the sleep and daytime functioning measures.

There were no significant findings for IIS. Three sleep variables, NAP (16% explained variance), SQR (5%), and TST (4%),were associated with BDI (Table A4.61). Higher NAP and lower SQR related to increased depression. As we have seen, increased TST was also related to increased depression.

Lower SQR and higher TST predicted STAI (Table A4.62). Jointly, they explained 13% of the variability in STAI, and SQR was more heavily weighted.

Summary. We identified eight significant findings for old men in the narrow normal sample (Table 4.20). NAP and SQR continue to be strongly related with daytime functioning. Paradoxical findings with TST persist.

Sleep and Daytime Functioning in the Old Women Group. Increased NAP predicted increased sleepiness on both of our sleepiness measures, ESS and SSS (Tables A4.63 and A4.64). NAP accounted for 13% and 18% of ESS and SSS variability, respectively.

NWAK explained 8% of the variability in FSS (Table A4.65). Increased NWAK was associated with increased FSS.

TABLE 4.20
Summary of Regression Analyses: Narrow Normal Sample, Old Men

| Sleep Measures | Measures of Daytime Functioning | | | | | |
	ESS	SSS	FSS	IIS	BDI	STAI
SOL						
NWAK						
WASO		+				
TST					+	+
SE						
SQR					−	−
NAP	+		+		+	

Note. Signs indicate the presence and direction of the relationship between the sleep and daytime functioning measures.

SOL explained 9% of the variability in IIS (Table A4.66). Increased SOL was associated with increased IIS.

SQR explained 8% of the variability in BDI (Table A4.67). Decreased SQR was associated with increased BDI. There were no significant findings for STAI.

Summary. For old women in the narrow normal sample, we encountered only five significant relationships between sleep and daytime functioning (Table 4.21). No more than one sleep variable was associated with any daytime measure.

Overall Summary of Regression Analyses Relating Sleep and Daytime Functioning

Across the broad and narrow normal samples, we identified eight unique subgroups and related sleep variables to each of six daytime functioning variables in each of these groups. In all, 48 regression procedures were performed. Table 4.22 reduces this large amount of information to counts of how many times a sleep measure was significantly related to a daytime measure.

TABLE 4.21
Summary of Regression Analyses: Narrow Normal Sample, Old Women

Sleep Measures	Measures of Daytime Functioning					
	ESS	SSS	FSS	IIS	BDI	STAI
SOL				+		
NWAK			+			
WASO						
TST						
SE						
SQR					−	
NAP	+	+				

Note. Signs indicate the presence and direction of the relationship between the sleep and daytime functioning measures.

TABLE 4.22

**Summary of All Regression Analyses: Count of Sleep Measures Related
to Daytime Functioning Measures**

Sleep Measures	Measures of Daytime Functioning						
	ESS	SSS	FSS	IIS	BDI	STAI	Total N
SOL	2			2			4
NWAK	1		1	1			3
WASO		1			2		3
TST			3	5	3	1	12
SE		2			1		3
SQR	3	4	5	6	7	7	32
NAP	7	6	3	5	3	1	25
Total N	13	11	14	19	16	9	82

The right column, labeled Total N, sums rows across daytime mea-sures and indicates which sleep measures were most often associated with daytime functioning. SQR (32 occurrences of 48 possibilities or 67% hit rate) and NAP (52% hit rate) are clearly separated from the pack. Without exception, lower SQR values and higher NAP minutes were associated with diminished daytime functioning, and these results were consistent with our expectations. The only other variable with a strong presence was TST (25% hit rate), and it was always positively cor-related with diminished daytime functioning. This outcome was unex-pected. SOL, NWAK, WASO, and SE were weakly related to daytime functioning.

Viewing the total count in the bottom row provides some index of which daytime measures were most closely tied to sleep experience. IIS was most strongly related to sleep (19 occurrences of 48 possibilities or 40% hit rate) and STAI least strongest (19%). No daytime functioning variable was strongly insulated from sleep, although the nature of the re-lationships remains a matter of conjecture. Chapter 7 presents further discussion of and hypotheses about the relationship between sleep and daytime functioning among normal sleepers (and those with insomnia).

4

Appendix

TABLE A4.1
Broad Normal Subset: Mean (SD) Sleep in Decade 20–29 Years of Age

Variable	Whole Sample					AA		CA	
	Total (n = 91)	Men (n = 45)	Women (n = 46)	AA (n = 37)	CA (n = 54)	Men (n = 17)	Women (n = 20)	Men (n = 28)	Women (n = 26)
SOL (min)	19.2 (12.5)	19.4 (9.5)	19.0 (15.0)	23.5 (17.2)	16.2 (6.6)	23.4 (11.8)	23.6 (21.1)	16.9 (6.9)	15.4 (6.3)
NWAK	1.1 (1.0)	0.9 (0.9)	1.3 (1.0)	1.1 (1.0)	1.1 (0.9)	0.7 (0.7)	1.5 (1.1)	1.0 (0.9)	1.2 (1.0)
WASO (min)	15.2 (18.3)	11.3 (11.9)	19.1 (22.4)	21.1 (24.3)	11.2 (11.2)	13.2 (12.7)	27.8 (29.7)	10.1 (11.5)	12.4 (11.0)
TST (min)	439.3 (66.7)	438.7 (68.1)	439.8 (66.0)	435.3 (94.6)	442.0 (38.0)	443.1 (106.4)	428.6 (85.6)	436.1 (28.7)	448.4 (45.6)
SE (%)	89.1 (6.0)	89.8 (4.9)	88.5 (7.0)	86.1 (7.4)	91.2 (3.8)	87.9 (6.0)	84.7 (8.2)	91.0 (3.7)	91.4 (4.0)
SQR	3.4 (0.5)	3.5 (0.5)	3.3 (0.5)	3.3 (0.6)	3.4 (0.5)	3.5 (0.6)	3.2 (0.6)	3.5 (0.5)	3.3 (0.5)
NAP (min)	14.2 (19.9)	12.7 (22.1)	15.6 (17.6)	24.2 (26.9)	7.3 (8.0)	25.1 (32.0)	23.4 (22.5)	5.2 (5.9)	9.6 (9.3)

TABLE A4.2
Broad Normal Subset: Mean (SD) Sleep in Decade 30–39 Years of Age

Variable	Whole Sample					AA		CA	
	Total (n = 97)	Men (n = 38)	Women (n = 59)	AA (n = 35)	CA (n = 62)	Men (n = 11)	Women (n = 24)	Men (n = 27)	Women (n = 35)
SOL (min)	17.9 (11.8)	15.5 (8.9)	19.5 (13.1)	23.9 (12.5)	14.5 (10.0)	20.1 (11.9)	25.7 (12.5)	13.6 (6.8)	15.2 (11.9)
NWAK	1.2 (0.8)	1.0 (0.8)	1.3 (0.8)	1.0 (0.8)	1.3 (0.9)	0.9 (0.9)	1.1 (0.7)	1.0 (0.8)	1.5 (0.9)
WASO (min)	15.8 (20.0)	13.8 (25.2)	17.2 (16.0)	20.5 (29.3)	13.2 (11.6)	22.6 (45.2)	19.5 (19.5)	10.2 (8.4)	15.6 (13.1)
TST (min)	413.6 (53.5)	410.4 (48.8)	415.6 (56.7)	401.5 (64.4)	420.4 (45.5)	389.7 (65.9)	407.0 (64.3)	418.9 (38.3)	421.6 (50.9)
SE (%)	88.6 (7.0)	90.0 (7.0)	87.7 (6.9)	85.2 (8.0)	90.5 (5.4)	85.6 (11.0)	85.0 (6.6)	91.8 (3.4)	89.6 (6.5)
SQR	3.5 (0.7)	3.6 (0.6)	3.4 (0.7)	3.3 (0.8)	3.6 (0.5)	3.5 (0.7)	3.2 (0.8)	3.7 (0.5)	3.5 (0.6)
NAP (min)	15.4 (19.1)	13.3 (17.2)	16.7 (20.3)	23.2 (24.9)	11.0 (13.2)	21.4 (22.0)	24.0 (26.5)	10.0 (14.0)	11.7 (12.8)

TABLE A4.3
Broad Normal Subset: Mean (SD) Sleep in Decade 40–49 Years of Age

Variable	Whole Sample					AA		CA	
	Total (n = 79)	Men (n = 43)	Women (n = 36)	AA (n = 25)	CA (n = 54)	Men (n = 16)	Women (n = 9)	Men (n = 27)	Women (n = 27)
SOL (min)	18.8 (15.0)	20.5 (16.7)	16.7 (12.8)	26.2 (20.6)	15.3 (10.1)	28.3 (23.0)	22.4 (16.1)	15.8 (9.2)	14.8 (11.1)
NWAK	1.2 (0.9)	1.2 (0.8)	1.3 (1.1)	1.3 (1.1)	1.2 (0.9)	1.2 (1.0)	1.5 (1.2)	1.3 (0.7)	1.2 (1.0)
WASO (min)	16.6 (18.4)	17.0 (20.5)	16.0 (15.8)	21.8 (26.6)	14.2 (12.6)	20.0 (29.2)	25.0 (22.5)	15.2 (13.3)	13.1 (11.9)
TST (min)	406.9 (51.9)	405.9 (57.3)	408.2 (45.3)	395.9 (65.3)	412.0 (44.1)	402.5 (68.1)	384.3 (62.2)	407.9 (51.1)	416.1 (36.3)
SE (%)	88.2 (9.0)	87.8 (9.7)	88.7 (8.2)	83.3 (12.8)	90.5 (5.4)	83.8 (13.6)	82.4 (11.8)	90.2 (5.3)	90.8 (5.5)
SQR	3.5 (0.6)	3.5 (0.6)	3.6 (0.6)	3.5 (0.6)	3.5 (0.6)	3.5 (0.5)	3.7 (0.8)	3.5 (0.7)	3.6 (0.6)
NAP (min)	11.3 (15.1)	11.4 (13.8)	11.3 (16.7)	17.7 (21.4)	8.4 (10.0)	13.9 (17.6)	24.4 (26.8)	9.9 (11.1)	6.9 (8.6)

TABLE A4.4
Broad Normal Subset: Mean (SD) Sleep in Decade 50–59 Years of Age

Variable	Whole Sample					AA		CA	
	Total (n = 92)	Men (n = 48)	Women (n = 44)	AA (n = 25)	CA (n = 67)	Men (n = 10)	Women (n = 15)	Men (n = 38)	Women (n = 29)
SOL (min)	17.6 (14.3)	16.6 (11.3)	18.8 (16.9)	23.1 (16.2)	15.6 (13.0)	21.2 (10.5)	24.4 (19.4)	15.3 (11.4)	15.9 (15.1)
NWAK	1.3 (1.0)	1.3 (1.1)	1.4 (0.9)	1.2 (1.0)	1.4 (1.0)	1.1 (0.9)	1.3 (1.0)	1.3 (1.1)	1.5 (0.8)
WASO (min)	13.0 (12.2)	12.1 (9.8)	13.9 (14.5)	14.7 (17.6)	12.3 (9.5)	10.9 (11.1)	17.3 (20.9)	12.5 (9.5)	12.1 (9.6)
TST (min)	415.1 (58.9)	408.5 (58.7)	422.2 (58.9)	407.7 (70.0)	417.8 (54.5)	386.2 (49.4)	422.1 (79.2)	414.4 (60.1)	422.3 (46.9)
SE (%)	89.6 (5.9)	90.3 (4.6)	88.9 (7.1)	87.3 (7.1)	90.5 (5.2)	88.8 (5.0)	86.3 (8.3)	90.8 (4.5)	90.2 (6.1)
SQR	3.6 (0.6)	3.6 (0.6)	3.5 (0.5)	3.6 (0.5)	3.6 (0.6)	3.7 (0.3)	3.6 (0.6)	3.6 (0.6)	3.5 (0.5)
NAP (min)	12.5 (18.3)	13.8 (22.0)	11.1 (13.4)	18.1 (16.9)	10.4 (18.5)	20.4 (14.9)	16.6 (18.5)	12.0 (23.3)	8.2 (9.0)

117

TABLE A4.5

Broad Normal Subset: Mean (SD) Sleep in Decade 60–69 Years of Age

Variable	Whole Sample			AA (n = 24)	CA (n = 65)	AA		CA	
	Total (n = 89)	Men (n = 47)	Women (n = 42)			Men (n = 9)	Women (n = 15)	Men (n = 38)	Women (n = 27)
SOL (min)	17.2 (12.3)	14.8 (10.6)	20.0 (13.5)	20.4 (12.3)	16.1 (12.1)	25.2 (16.8)	17.5 (7.9)	12.3 (6.8)	21.4 (15.7)
NWAK	1.5 (1.0)	1.6 (1.0)	1.4 (0.9)	1.2 (0.9)	1.6 (1.0)	1.5 (0.9)	1.0 (0.9)	1.6 (1.0)	1.5 (0.9)
WASO (min)	22.6 (23.2)	21.6 (23.3)	23.6 (23.4)	23.3 (22.1)	22.3 (23.8)	24.1 (20.0)	22.9 (24.0)	21.0 (24.2)	24.0 (23.5)
TST (min)	428.7 (61.1)	434.8 (65.6)	421.8 (55.5)	417.5 (46.1)	432.8 (65.6)	416.4 (54.4)	418.2 (42.4)	439.2 (67.9)	423.8 (62.3)
SE (%)	88.0 (7.5)	89.3 (6.3)	86.6 (8.4)	85.8 (6.3)	88.9 (7.7)	85.7 (4.8)	85.9 (7.1)	90.2 (6.4)	87.0 (9.1)
SQR	3.7 (0.7)	3.6 (0.7)	3.8 (0.7)	3.9 (0.7)	3.6 (0.7)	3.7 (0.9)	4.0 (0.6)	3.6 (0.6)	3.7 (0.7)
NAP (min)	18.3 (25.7)	18.9 (20.4)	17.6 (30.8)	14.6 (16.4)	19.6 (28.4)	14.2 (17.1)	14.8 (16.5)	20.0 (21.2)	19.1 (36.6)

TABLE A4.6
Broad Normal Subset: Mean (SD) Sleep in Decade 70–79 Years of Age

Variable	Whole Sample					AA		CA	
	Total (n = 80)	Men (n = 38)	Women (n = 42)	AA (n = 12)	CA (n = 68)	Men (n = 5)	Women (n = 7)	Men (n = 33)	Women (n = 35)
SOL (min)	20.1 (16.3)	14.8 (12.9)	24.8 (17.8)	28.1 (18.8)	18.7 (15.6)	25.8 (25.8)	29.7 (13.9)	13.2 (9.4)	23.8 (18.4)
NWAK	1.6 (0.9)	1.5 (0.9)	1.7 (0.9)	1.5 (1.3)	1.6 (0.8)	1.2 (1.0)	1.8 (1.5)	1.5 (0.9)	1.7 (0.7)
WASO (min)	21.7 (19.2)	20.6 (24.2)	22.7 (13.5)	22.8 (16.8)	21.5 (19.7)	9.3 (8.2)	32.5 (14.6)	22.3 (25.5)	20.8 (12.6)
TST (min)	428.7 (63.6)	420.7 (72.3)	435.9 (54.3)	459.6 (61.9)	423.2 (62.7)	465.2 (77.6)	455.7 (54.4)	414.0 (70.3)	431.9 (54.2)
SE (%)	87.8 (6.0)	89.0 (6.3)	86.7 (5.6)	86.0 (7.4)	88.1 (5.8)	90.3 (6.9)	82.9 (6.4)	88.8 (6.3)	87.4 (5.2)
SQR	3.6 (0.7)	3.6 (0.6)	3.5 (0.7)	3.5 (0.7)	3.6 (0.7)	3.8 (0.9)	3.4 (0.4)	3.6 (0.6)	3.5 (0.8)
NAP (min)	19.3 (24.2)	23.5 (28.3)	15.4 (19.3)	26.9 (25.4)	17.9 (23.9)	31.7 (26.5)	23.4 (26.1)	22.3 (28.8)	13.8 (17.7)

TABLE A4.7
Broad Normal Subset: Mean (SD) Sleep in Decade 80-89+ Years of Age

Variable	Whole Sample					AA		CA	
	Total (n = 65)	Men (n = 35)	Women (n = 30)	AA (n = 20)	CA (n = 45)	Men (n = 11)	Women (n = 9)	Men (n = 24)	Women (n = 21)
SOL (min)	20.5 (11.1)	18.2 (10.2)	23.2 (11.7)	23.1 (9.9)	19.3 (11.5)	20.3 (9.5)	26.4 (9.9)	17.2 (10.6)	21.8 (12.3)
NWAK	1.8 (1.1)	1.7 (1.2)	1.9 (1.0)	1.5 (1.2)	2.0 (1.1)	0.9 (0.9)	2.2 (1.2)	2.1 (1.2)	1.8 (0.9)
WASO (min)	26.0 (23.8)	19.7 (15.5)	33.3 (29.3)	20.4 (17.2)	28.4 (25.9)	13.3 (12.5)	29.1 (18.9)	22.6 (16.1)	35.1 (33.1)
TST (min)	461.8 (71.0)	465.6 (56.8)	457.3 (85.5)	494.4 (80.8)	447.3 (61.8)	512.2 (58.6)	472.6 (101.1)	444.3 (42.1)	450.7 (79.7)
SE (%)	87.0 (7.2)	89.5 (5.7)	84.0 (7.7)	87.0 (7.5)	87.0 (7.1)	90.8 (3.6)	82.4 (8.6)	89.0 (6.4)	84.7 (7.4)
SQR	3.7 (0.7)	3.7 (0.8)	3.7 (0.5)	3.6 (0.6)	3.7 (0.7)	3.7 (0.7)	3.5 (0.5)	3.7 (0.8)	3.8 (0.5)
NAP (min)	24.2 (21.2)	21.7 (20.6)	27.2 (21.9)	38.2 (22.8)	18.0 (17.4)	29.7 (20.9)	48.6 (21.7)	18.1 (19.8)	18.0 (14.6)

TABLE A4.8

Narrow Normal Subset: Mean (SD) Sleep in Decade 20–29 Years of Age

Variable	Whole Sample					AA		CA	
	Total (n = 68)	Men (n = 35)	Women (n = 33)	AA (n = 21)	CA (n = 47)	Men (n = 11)	Women (n = 10)	Men (n = 24)	Women (n = 23)
SOL (min)	15.9 (5.9)	16.9 (6.3)	14.9 (5.3)	17.9 (5.6)	15.0 (5.8)	20.2 (5.6)	15.4 (4.7)	15.4 (6.1)	14.6 (5.6)
NWAK	0.9 (0.8)	0.7 (0.7)	1.1 (0.9)	0.8 (0.7)	1.0 (0.9)	0.5 (0.5)	1.0 (0.8)	0.8 (0.8)	1.2 (1.0)
WASO (min)	9.3 (7.9)	7.0 (5.5)	11.7 (9.4)	10.3 (8.4)	8.9 (7.7)	7.7 (6.2)	13.1 (9.8)	6.7 (5.2)	11.1 (9.3)
TST (min)	445.6 (48.7)	439.6 (32.7)	452.1 (61.2)	450.0 (65.6)	443.7 (39.6)	441.6 (39.9)	459.3 (87.3)	438.6 (29.8)	448.9 (47.9)
SE (%)	91.5 (3.4)	91.5 (3.2)	91.4 (3.7)	90.4 (3.7)	91.9 (3.2)	90.7 (3.6)	90.0 (4.0)	91.8 (3.0)	92.1 (3.5)
SQR	3.5 (0.5)	3.5 (0.5)	3.5 (0.5)	3.6 (0.5)	3.5 (0.5)	3.5 (0.5)	3.6 (0.6)	3.6 (0.5)	3.4 (0.5)
NAP (min)	12.3 (19.1)	11.7 (20.6)	12.8 (17.7)	23.3 (30.0)	7.3 (7.7)	25.4 (32.4)	21.0 (28.6)	5.4 (6.1)	9.3 (8.9)

TABLE A4.9
Narrow Normal Subset: Mean (SD) Sleep in Decade 30–39 Years of Age

Variable	Whole Sample					AA		CA	
	Total (n = 64)	Men (n = 30)	Women (n = 34)	AA (n = 16)	CA (n = 48)	Men (n = 7)	Women (n = 9)	Men (n = 23)	Women (n = 25)
SOL (min)	13.9 (7.5)	13.7 (7.1)	14.0 (8.0)	17.6 (8.6)	12.6 (6.8)	15.3 (8.7)	19.3 (8.7)	13.2 (6.8)	12.1 (6.9)
NWAK	1.0 (0.7)	0.8 (0.7)	1.2 (0.7)	0.6 (0.5)	1.2 (0.7)	0.4 (0.4)	0.8 (0.5)	1.0 (0.7)	1.3 (0.8)
WASO (min)	9.8 (7.8)	8.8 (8.4)	10.7 (7.1)	7.7 (8.7)	10.5 (7.4)	4.1 (4.1)	10.5 (10.4)	10.2 (8.9)	10.7 (5.8)
TST (min)	424.2 (46.5)	418.6 (46.2)	429.2 (46.9)	416.8 (61.0)	426.7 (41.1)	411.7 (63.3)	420.8 (62.7)	420.7 (41.3)	432.2 (41.0)
SE (%)	91.3 (4.0)	91.5 (4.6)	91.1 (3.4)	89.5 (5.5)	91.9 (3.2)	90.6 (7.3)	88.6 (3.8)	91.7 (3.7)	92.0 (2.9)
SQR	3.7 (0.6)	3.8 (0.6)	3.6 (0.6)	3.5 (0.8)	3.7 (0.5)	3.8 (0.8)	3.3 (0.8)	3.8 (0.5)	3.7 (0.4)
NAP (min)	11.5 (13.1)	8.8 (12.5)	14.0 (13.4)	16.2 (13.5)	10.0 (12.8)	11.6 (10.3)	19.7 (15.2)	7.9 (13.2)	11.9 (12.3)

TABLE A4.10
Narrow Normal Subset: Mean (SD) Sleep in Decade 40–49 Years of Age

Variable	Whole Sample					AA		CA	
	Total (n = 59)	Men (n = 35)	Women (n = 24)	AA (n = 14)	CA (n = 45)	Men (n = 11)	Women (n = 3)	Men (n = 24)	Women (n = 21)
SOL (min)	13.6 (7.6)	14.8 (8.1)	11.9 (6.6)	15.8 (7.1)	12.9 (7.7)	16.2 (8.0)	14.5 (2.7)	14.2 (8.2)	11.5 (6.9)
NWAK	1.1 (0.8)	1.1 (0.8)	1.2 (0.9)	1.0 (0.8)	1.2 (0.8)	0.8 (0.8)	1.7 (0.7)	1.3 (0.8)	1.1 (0.9)
WASO (min)	11.4 (10.0)	11.7 (10.8)	10.9 (9.0)	10.2 (9.4)	11.8 (10.3)	8.9 (10.0)	14.9 (5.6)	13.0 (11.1)	10.4 (9.3)
TST (min)	414.7 (46.2)	412.4 (50.2)	418.0 (40.4)	415.1 (64.2)	414.6 (39.9)	422.2 (63.0)	388.9 (74.8)	407.9 (43.9)	422.2 (34.2)
SE (%)	91.2 (4.9)	90.7 (5.0)	91.9 (4.8)	89.9 (5.6)	91.6 (4.7)	89.9 (6.0)	89.9 (4.7)	91.0 (4.5)	92.2 (4.9)
SQR	3.6 (0.6)	3.5 (0.6)	3.7 (0.6)	3.7 (C.4)	3.5 (0.7)	3.6 (0.4)	4.0 (0.0)	3.4 (0.7)	3.6 (0.7)
NAP (min)	8.3 (11.4)	10.2 (13.1)	5.5 (7.7)	12.9 (15.5)	6.8 (9.5)	13.7 (17.1)	10.0 (8.7)	8.6 (10.8)	4.8 (7.6)

TABLE A4.11

Narrow Normal Subset: Mean (SD) Sleep in Decade 50–59 Years of Age

| | Whole Sample | | | | | AA | | CA | |
	Total (n = 60)	Men (n = 32)	Women (n = 28)	AA (n = 15)	CA (n = 45)	Men (n = 5)	Women (n = 10)	Men (n = 27)	Women (n = 18)
Variable									
SOL (min)	13.3 (8.0)	13.2 (8.5)	13.4 (7.5)	15.6 (7.7)	12.5 (8.0)	13.4 (7.1)	16.6 (8.2)	13.2 (8.8)	11.6 (6.7)
NWAK	1.1 (1.0)	1.0 (1.0)	1.2 (0.9)	0.9 (1.0)	1.2 (1.0)	0.7 (0.7)	1.1 (1.1)	1.1 (1.1)	1.3 (0.8)
WASO (min)	8.9 (7.6)	8.8 (7.8)	8.9 (7.6)	6.9 (8.6)	9.6 (7.3)	3.8 (3.0)	8.4 (10.2)	9.8 (8.1)	9.2 (6.0)
TST (min)	414.1 (63.2)	411.4 (66.5)	417.2 (60.2)	405.9 (69.9)	416.9 (61.3)	388.5 (58.9)	414.6 (76.2)	415.6 (68.0)	418.7 (51.6)
SE (%)	91.3 (4.6)	91.7 (4.3)	90.9 (4.8)	90.7 (4.3)	91.5 (4.7)	92.5 (4.5)	89.7 (4.0)	91.5 (4.4)	91.6 (5.2)
SQR	3.8 (0.5)	3.8 (0.6)	3.7 (0.5)	3.8 (0.5)	3.7 (0.6)	3.9 (0.1)	3.8 (0.6)	3.8 (0.6)	3.6 (0.4)
NAP (min)	12.5 (21.1)	14.3 (26.0)	10.5 (13.8)	17.8 (18.9)	10.8 (21.7)	20.3 (18.0)	16.6 (20.2)	13.2 (27.4)	7.1 (7.2)

TABLE A4.12
Narrow Normal Subset: Mean (SD) Sleep in Decade 60–69 Years of Age

Variable	Whole Sample					AA		CA	
	Total (n = 58)	Men (n = 30)	Women (n = 28)	AA (n = 15)	CA (n = 43)	Men (n = 5)	Women (n = 10)	Men (n = 25)	Women (n = 18)
SOL (min)	12.8 (6.3)	11.5 (5.6)	14.1 (6.8)	15.7 (4.8)	11.8 (6.5)	16.3 (4.0)	15.4 (5.4)	10.5 (5.4)	13.5 (7.6)
NWAK	1.3 (0.9)	1.6 (1.0)	1.0 (0.7)	1.1 (0.9)	1.4 (0.9)	1.9 (0.8)	0.8 (0.6)	1.6 (1.0)	1.2 (0.7)
WASO (min)	11.6 (9.7)	11.7 (8.4)	11.6 (11.0)	10.6 (9.1)	12.0 (10.0)	15.3 (10.6)	8.2 (7.7)	11.0 (8.0)	13.4 (12.3)
TST (min)	438.6 (54.1)	439.4 (63.2)	437.7 (43.3)	414.7 (40.7)	447.0 (56.0)	398.4 (40.7)	422.8 (40.3)	447.7 (64.3)	446.0 (43.8)
SE (%)	91.4 (4.8)	91.9 (4.6)	90.9 (5.0)	88.6 (5.4)	92.4 (4.2)	87.6 (4.8)	89.1 (5.8)	92.8 (4.1)	91.9 (4.4)
SQR	3.9 (0.6)	3.9 (0.6)	4.0 (0.6)	4.0 (0.7)	3.9 (0.6)	4.0 (1.1)	3.9 (0.6)	3.8 (0.5)	4.0 (0.7)
NAP (min)	13.3 (15.6)	16.9 (17.0)	9.5 (13.1)	12.6 (15.7)	13.6 (15.7)	11.7 (9.3)	13.0 (18.5)	18.0 (18.1)	7.6 (8.9)

TABLE A4.13
Narrow Normal Subset: Mean (SD) Sleep in Decade 70–79 Years of Age

Variable	Whole Sample					AA		CA	
	Total (n = 47)	Men (n = 26)	Women (n = 21)	AA (n = 6)	CA (n = 41)	Men (n = 4)	Women (n = 2)	Men (n = 22)	Women (n = 19)
SOL (min)	15.5 (15.3)	12.7 (10.9)	19.0 (19.2)	18.8 (19.7)	15.0 (14.8)	19.7 (25.4)	16.9 (0.5)	11.4 (6.1)	19.3 (20.3)
NWAK	1.5 (0.9)	1.3 (1.0)	1.6 (0.8)	1.4 (1.0)	1.5 (0.9)	1.2 (1.2)	1.9 (0.8)	1.4 (1.0)	1.6 (0.8)
WASO (min)	13.4 (10.2)	10.3 (6.5)	17.3 (12.6)	15.5 (19.4)	13.1 (8.5)	5.8 (2.8)	34.9 (27.0)	11.1 (6.7)	15.5 (9.9)
TST (min)	436.6 (65.2)	424.0 (78.1)	452.2 (41.4)	467.6 (65.8)	432.1 (64.7)	480.6 (80.3)	441.6 (17.3)	413.7 (74.9)	453.3 (43.3)
SE (%)	90.7 (4.1)	91.8 (3.4)	89.4 (4.7)	90.5 (5.7)	90.8 (3.9)	93.1 (3.6)	85.3 (6.6)	91.5 (3.3)	89.8 (4.5)
SQR	3.6 (0.7)	3.7 (0.7)	3.6 (0.7)	3.6 (0.8)	3.7 (0.7)	3.7 (1.0)	3.4 (0.1)	3.7 (0.7)	3.6 (0.8)
NAP (min)	18.4 (18.8)	23.9 (20.5)	11.6 (14.1)	32.5 (21.2)	16.3 (17.8)	39.6 (22.8)	18.3 (9.0)	21.1 (19.3)	10.8 (14.5)

TABLE A4.14
Narrow Normal Subset: Mean (SD) Sleep in Decade 80–89+ Years of Age

Variable	Whole Sample					AA		CA	
	Total (n = 36)	Men (n = 24)	Women (n = 12)	AA (n = 10)	CA (n = 26)	Men (n = 8)	Women (n = 2)	Men (n = 16)	Women (n = 10)
SOL (min)	15.4 (8.7)	14.8 (8.4)	16.7 (9.6)	18.9 (9.8)	14.1 (8.1)	19.4 (10.4)	16.6 (9.3)	12.5 (6.5)	16.7 (10.1)
NWAK	1.4 (1.0)	1.3 (0.9)	1.6 (1.1)	1.0 (1.3)	1.6 (0.8)	0.6 (0.7)	2.7 (2.2)	1.7 (0.8)	1.3 (0.8)
WASO (min)	13.6 (10.1)	12.9 (9.8)	15.0 (11.0)	10.3 (9.7)	14.9 (10.2)	8.8 (10.1)	16.4 (6.1)	14.9 (9.3)	14.8 (11.9)
TST (min)	475.0 (77.0)	470.5 (53.0)	483.9 (113.3)	509.0 (98.0)	461.9 (64.7)	503.2 (62.4)	532.3 (240.7)	454.2 (40.5)	474.2 (92.9)
SE (%)	91.1 (3.8)	91.7 (3.9)	89.9 (3.2)	91.4 (3.2)	91.0 (4.0)	91.7 (3.6)	90.6 (0.7)	91.7 (4.2)	89.8 (3.5)
SQR	4.0 (0.5)	3.9 (0.6)	4.0 (0.4)	3.9 (0.6)	4.0 (0.5)	3.9 (0.7)	3.9 (0.3)	3.9 (0.6)	4.0 (0.4)
NAP (min)	20.5 (18.6)	17.8 (17.4)	26.0 (20.6)	31.0 (23.1)	16.5 (15.2)	24.4 (21.0)	57.1 (2.5)	14.4 (14.9)	19.7 (16.0)

128

TABLE A4.15
Full Sample: Mean (SD) Sleep in Decade 20–29 Years of Age

Variable	Whole Sample[a]					AA		CA	
	Total (n = 105)	Men (n = 53)	Women (n = 52)	AA (n = 41)	CA (n = 61)	Men (n = 18)	Women (n = 23)	Men (n = 32)	Women (n = 29)
SOL (min)	21.1 (13.9)	20.1 (10.3)	22.1 (16.9)	25.4 (17.9)	18.6 (9.7)	23.3 (11.5)	27.0 (21.8)	19.0 (9.2)	18.2 (10.5)
NWAK	1.1 (1.0)	0.9 (0.9)	1.3 (1.0)	1.1 (1.0)	1.1 (1.0)	0.7 (0.7)	1.5 (1.1)	1.1 (1.0)	1.2 (1.0)
WASO (min)	14.9 (17.8)	11.1 (11.5)	18.8 (22.0)	19.9 (23.4)	12.1 (12.4)	12.7 (12.5)	25.5 (28.3)	10.9 (11.4)	13.4 (13.6)
TST (min)	435.4 (66.7)	437.2 (65.5)	433.5 (68.4)	431.1 (91.4)	437.1 (44.2)	438.9 (104.8)	425.1 (81.4)	434.2 (29.7)	440.2 (56.5)
SE (%)	88.7 (6.1)	89.6 (5.2)	87.8 (6.9)	86.1 (7.1)	90.2 (4.8)	88.1 (5.9)	84.6 (7.7)	90.1 (4.7)	90.3 (5.1)
SQR	3.3 (0.6)	3.4 (0.6)	3.3 (0.6)	3.3 (0.6)	3.4 (0.5)	3.4 (0.6)	3.2 (0.6)	3.5 (0.5)	3.4 (0.5)
NAP (min)	14.9 (20.1)	13.7 (22.7)	16.1 (17.2)	22.7 (26.0)	8.8 (9.7)	23.7 (31.6)	21.9 (21.4)	6.3 (7.1)	11.6 (11.4)

[a]These columns include the 10 subjects who did not code for AA or CA: 7 individuals of Asian decent, 1 of Hispanic decent, and 2 with missing ethnicity data.

TABLE A4.16

Full Sample: Mean (SD) Sleep in Decade 30–39 Years of Age

Variable	Whole Sample[a]					AA		CA	
	Total (n = 123)	Men (n = 54)	Women (n = 69)	AA (n = 47)	CA (n = 72)	Men (n = 18)	Women (n = 29)	Men (n = 33)	Women (n = 39)
SOL (min)	20.9 (14.5)	20.3 (14.4)	21.3 (14.6)	28.1 (16.0)	16.5 (11.7)	28.7 (17.5)	27.8 (15.4)	16.5 (11.0)	16.6 (12.4)
NWAK	1.3 (1.0)	1.2 (1.0)	1.4 (1.0)	1.2 (1.0)	1.4 (1.0)	1.2 (1.3)	1.1 (0.7)	1.2 (0.9)	1.6 (1.2)
WASO (min)	22.1 (30.7)	23.7 (40.4)	20.8 (20.5)	29.6 (43.8)	17.8 (17.7)	39.1 (64.4)	23.7 (23.4)	16.6 (17.1)	18.9 (18.4)
TST (min)	410.7 (58.2)	407.1 (56.4)	413.5 (59.8)	398.8 (67.0)	416.2 (50.8)	390.5 (68.3)	404.0 (66.9)	412.5 (47.3)	419.3 (54.1)
SE (%)	86.8 (8.2)	87.0 (9.3)	86.6 (7.3)	82.9 (9.4)	89.2 (6.4)	81.7 (12.5)	83.6 (7.0)	89.7 (5.8)	88.7 (6.9)
SQR	3.4 (0.7)	3.5 (0.6)	3.3 (0.7)	3.2 (0.8)	3.5 (0.6)	3.4 (0.7)	3.1 (0.8)	3.5 (0.6)	3.4 (0.7)
NAP (min)	16.7 (19.4)	14.6 (18.1)	18.4 (20.4)	25.0 (24.9)	11.7 (12.9)	22.3 (23.9)	26.7 (25.8)	11.0 (13.3)	12.2 (12.8)

[a]These columns include the 10 subjects who did not code for AA or CA: 7 individuals of Asian decent, 1 of Hispanic decent, and 2 with missing ethnicity data.

TABLE A4.17

Full Sample: Mean (SD) Sleep in Decade 40–49 Years of Age

| | Whole Sample[a] | | | | | AA | | CA | |
Variable	Total (n = 105)	Men (n = 54)	Women (n = 51)	AA (n = 34)	CA (n = 71)	Men (n = 18)	Women (n = 16)	Men (n = 36)	Women (n = 35)
SOL (min)	21.9 (18.8)	22.0 (18.9)	21.7 (18.9)	31.6 (25.0)	17.2 (12.8)	32.3 (25.0)	30.8 (25.7)	16.9 (12.4)	17.6 (13.3)
NWAK	1.4 (1.1)	1.4 (0.9)	1.4 (1.3)	1.3 (1.1)	1.4 (1.1)	1.2 (1.0)	1.4 (1.2)	1.5 (0.9)	1.4 (1.3)
WASO (min)	21.4 (24.3)	21.9 (26.2)	20.9 (22.3)	27.8 (32.6)	18.4 (18.5)	26.6 (33.5)	29.2 (32.7)	19.6 (21.8)	17.1 (14.5)
TST (min)	404.9 (65.1)	401.4 (57.8)	408.7 (72.4)	394.1 (67.8)	410.1 (63.6)	398.2 (65.1)	389.5 (72.6)	402.9 (54.7)	417.5 (71.6)
SE (%)	86.5 (10.2)	86.3 (10.6)	86.7 (9.9)	81.6 (13.5)	88.8 (7.3)	82.2 (13.7)	81.0 (13.7)	88.4 (8.2)	89.2 (6.3)
SQR	3.4 (0.7)	3.4 (0.6)	3.4 (0.7)	3.3 (0.7)	3.4 (0.6)	3.3 (0.6)	3.3 (0.9)	3.4 (0.7)	3.4 (0.6)
NAP (min)	13.7 (18.7)	12.8 (17.6)	14.5 (19.9)	22.2 (27.4)	9.6 (10.6)	18.1 (25.2)	26.8 (29.8)	10.2 (11.7)	8.9 (9.4)

[a]These columns include the 10 subjects who did not code for AA or CA: 7 individuals of Asian decent, 1 of Hispanic decent, and 2 with missing ethnicity data.

TABLE A4.18
Full Sample: Mean (SD) Sleep in Decade 50–59 Years of Age

Variable	Whole Sample[a]					AA		CA	
	Total (n = 117)	Men (n = 59)	Women (n = 58)	AA (n = 32)	CA (n = 84)	Men (n = 12)	Women (n = 20)	Men (n = 46)	Women (n = 38)
SOL (min)	21.0 (16.7)	17.7 (12.2)	24.3 (19.9)	29.0 (19.5)	18.0 (14.7)	23.7 (11.1)	32.2 (22.8)	16.1 (12.3)	20.2 (17.0)
NWAK	1.4 (1.0)	1.4 (1.1)	1.5 (1.0)	1.3 (1.3)	1.5 (1.1)	1.2 (0.9)	1.4 (1.0)	1.4 (1.1)	1.6 (1.0)
WASO (min)	17.0 (18.1)	14.3 (12.4)	19.7 (22.3)	20.6 (24.4)	15.7 (15.1)	15.4 (14.9)	23.7 (28.6)	14.2 (11.9)	17.6 (18.2)
TST (min)	405.8 (62.7)	403.9 (63.2)	407.7 (62.7)	390.7 (75.1)	411.4 (57.2)	370.9 (57.2)	402.6 (83.1)	412.2 (63.0)	410.4 (49.9)
SE (%)	87.7 (7.8)	89.3 (6.1)	86.0 (9.0)	84.2 (9.3)	89.0 (6.9)	86.7 (6.7)	82.8 (10.4)	90.0 (5.9)	87.8 (7.8)
SQR	3.4 (0.6)	3.5 (0.7)	3.4 (0.6)	3.5 (0.6)	3.4 (0.7)	3.5 (0.5)	3.4 (0.7)	3.5 (0.7)	3.3 (0.6)
NAP (min)	14.1 (19.5)	13.6 (21.0)	14.6 (18.1)	20.8 (18.4)	11.7 (19.5)	20.2 (14.4)	21.2 (20.8)	12.2 (22.3)	11.2 (15.7)

[a]These columns include the 10 subjects who did not code for AA or CA: 7 individuals of Asian decent, 1 of Hispanic decent, and 2 with missing ethnicity data.

TABLE A4.19

Full Sample: Mean (SD) Sleep in Decade 60–69 Years of Age

Variable	Whole Sample[a]			AA		AA		CA	
	Total (n = 107)	Men (n = 55)	Women (n = 52)	AA (n = 27)	CA (n = 79)	Men (n = 9)	Women (n = 18)	Men (n = 45)	Women (n = 34)
SOL (min)	20.9 (15.5)	16.8 (12.1)	25.2 (17.5)	22.7 (13.3)	20.3 (16.3)	25.2 (16.8)	21.4 (11.5)	15.0 (10.5)	27.3 (19.7)
NWAK	1.6 (1.0)	1.7 (1.0)	1.6 (1.0)	1.4 (1.0)	1.7 (1.0)	1.5 (0.9)	1.3 (1.0)	1.7 (1.0)	1.7 (1.0)
WASO (min)	25.8 (23.8)	23.7 (23.4)	27.9 (24.2)	28.1 (25.0)	25.1 (23.6)	24.1 (20.0)	30.1 (27.4)	23.9 (24.4)	26.8 (22.7)
TST (min)	424.5 (62.8)	430.8 (65.7)	417.8 (59.6)	409.5 (52.1)	429.9 (65.9)	416.4 (54.4)	406.1 (52.1)	434.4 (68.4)	424.0 (63.0)
SE (%)	86.7 (8.0)	88.5 (6.5)	84.8 (8.9)	84.2 (7.7)	87.5 (7.9)	85.7 (4.8)	83.4 (8.9)	89.0 (6.7)	85.5 (9.0)
SQR	3.6 (0.7)	3.5 (0.7)	3.7 (0.8)	3.8 (0.7)	3.5 (0.7)	3.7 (0.9)	3.9 (0.6)	3.5 (0.6)	3.6 (0.8)
NAP (min)	18.1 (24.2)	19.2 (19.5)	17.0 (28.5)	15.7 (16.2)	19.1 (26.6)	14.2 (17.1)	16.5 (16.2)	20.4 (20.1)	17.3 (33.5)

[a]These columns include the 10 subjects who did not code for AA or CA: 7 individuals of Asian decent, 1 of Hispanic decent, and 2 with missing ethnicity data.

TABLE A4.20
Full Sample: Mean (SD) Sleep in Decade 70–79 Years of Age

Variable	Whole Sample[a]			AA (n = 16)	CA (n = 95)	AA		CA	
	Total (n = 112)	Men (n = 54)	Women (n = 58)			Men (n = 6)	Women (n = 10)	Men (n = 47)	Women (n = 48)
SOL (min)	24.8 (20.4)	20.7 (20.9)	28.6 (19.4)	28.8 (17.5)	24.0 (20.9)	28.3 (23.9)	29.1 (13.9)	19.4 (20.6)	28.5 (20.4)
NWAK	1.9 (1.1)	1.8 (1.1)	1.9 (1.0)	1.6 (1.1)	1.9 (1.0)	1.3 (0.9)	1.9 (1.2)	1.8 (1.1)	1.9 (1.0)
WASO (min)	36.0 (37.1)	33.7 (32.9)	38.2 (40.8)	47.6 (60.8)	33.9 (31.7)	23.5 (35.6)	62.0 (69.6)	34.5 (32.9)	33.3 (30.7)
TST (min)	409.5 (74.6)	405.7 (79.7)	413.0 (70.0)	419.3 (97.1)	408.0 (71.0)	449.1 (79.8)	401.4 (106.0)	400.5 (79.7)	415.4 (61.3)
SE (%)	83.2 (10.8)	84.2 (11.2)	82.3 (10.5)	79.9 (14.4)	83.8 (10.1)	86.5 (11.3)	75.9 (15.1)	84.0 (11.3)	83.6 (9.0)
SQR	3.3 (0.7)	3.4 (0.7)	3.3 (0.7)	3.3 (0.7)	3.3 (0.7)	3.5 (0.9)	3.1 (0.6)	3.4 (0.7)	3.3 (0.8)
NAP (min)	20.8 (25.4)	25.6 (30.3)	16.4 (19.1)	30.5 (23.6)	19.3 (25.6)	34.2 (24.5)	28.3 (24.1)	24.9 (31.2)	13.9 (17.2)

[a]These columns include the 10 subjects who did not code for AA or CA: 7 individuals of Asian decent, 1 of Hispanic decent, and 2 with missing ethnicity data.

TABLE A4.21

Full Sample: Mean (SD) Sleep in Decade 80–89+ Years of Age

Variable	Whole Sample[a]			AA (n = 26)	CA (n = 77)	AA		CA	
	Total (n = 103)	Men (n = 52)	Women (n = 51)			Men (n = 12)	Women (n = 14)	Men (n = 40)	Women (n = 37)
SOL (min)	31.0 (26.3)	22.3 (14.3)	39.9 (32.3)	27.6 (13.1)	32.2 (29.4)	22.3 (11.3)	32.2 (13.3)	22.3 (15.2)	42.9 (36.8)
NWAK	2.0 (1.1)	2.0 (1.2)	2.1 (1.1)	1.8 (1.3)	2.1 (1.1)	1.1 (1.1)	2.4 (1.2)	2.2 (1.2)	1.9 (1.0)
WASO (min)	36.9 (33.7)	31.0 (27.2)	43.0 (38.6)	39.3 (48.3)	36.1 (27.6)	20.4 (27.1)	55.5 (57.0)	34.1 (26.8)	38.3 (28.5)
TST (min)	448.6 (85.4)	459.4 (78.0)	437.7 (91.9)	464.8 (101.2)	443.2 (79.4)	489.8 (95.6)	443.3 (104.3)	450.2 (70.8)	435.6 (88.2)
SE (%)	82.6 (10.4)	86.3 (8.4)	78.8 (11.1)	81.5 (13.1)	82.9 (9.5)	88.1 (9.9)	75.9 (13.2)	85.7 (7.9)	79.9 (10.1)
SQR	3.5 (0.7)	3.4 (0.8)	3.5 (0.6)	3.3 (0.8)	3.5 (0.7)	3.6 (0.9)	3.1 (0.7)	3.4 (0.8)	3.6 (0.6)
NAP (min)	31.1 (32.0)	32.4 (37.4)	29.8 (25.5)	39.9 (26.9)	28.2 (33.1)	36.1 (29.7)	43.1 (24.9)	31.4 (39.7)	24.7 (24.2)

[a]These columns include the 10 subjects who did not code for AA or CA: 7 individuals of Asian decent, 1 of Hispanic decent, and 2 with missing ethnicity data.

TABLE A4.22
Broad Normal Sample: Stepwise Regression of the Epworth Sleepiness Scale on Sleep Variables Among Young Adults (N = 359)

Variable	B	SE B	β	ΔR^2
Step 1				
SQR	−1.45	0.36	−0.21	.04
Step 2				
NAP	0.04	0.01	0.17	.03
Step 3				
SOL	−0.05	0.01	−0.17	.03
Step 4				
NWAK	0.48	0.23	0.11	.01

Note. Significance criterion for variable entry is $p < .05$. Cumulative $R^2 = .11$.

TABLE A4.23
Broad Normal Sample: Stepwise Regression of the Stanford Sleepiness Scale on Sleep Variables Among Young Adults (N = 359)

Variable	B	SE B	β	ΔR^2
Step 1				
SQR	−0.60	0.13	−0.25	.06
Step 2				
NAP	0.01	0.00	0.14	.02

Note. Significance criterion for variable entry is $p < .05$. Cumulative $R^2 = .08$.

TABLE A4.24
Broad Normal Sample: Stepwise Regression of the Fatigue Severity Scale on Sleep Variables Among Young Adults ($N = 359$)

Variable	B	SE B	β	ΔR^2
Step 1				
SQR	−0.45	0.10	−0.24	.06

Note. Significance criterion for variable entry is $p < .05$.

TABLE A4.25
Broad Normal Sample: Stepwise Regression of the Insomnia Impact Scale on Sleep Variables Among Young Adults ($N = 359$)

Variable	B	SE B	β	ΔR^2
Step 1				
SQR	−12.97	1.81	−0.36	.13
Step 2				
TST	0.06	0.02	0.16	.02
Step 3				
NAP	0.19	0.06	0.16	.02

Note. Significance criterion for variable entry is $p < .05$. Cumulative $R^2 = .17$.

TABLE A4.26
Broad Normal Sample: Stepwise Regression of the Beck Depression Inventory on Sleep Variables Among Young Adults ($N = 359$)

Variable	B	SE B	β	ΔR^2
Step 1				
SQR	−3.51	0.57	−0.31	.10
Step 2				
WASO	0.06	0.02	0.16	.02

Note. Significance criterion for variable entry is $p < .05$. Cumulative $R^2 = .12$.

136

TABLE A4.27
Broad Normal Sample: Stepwise Regression of the State-Trait Anxiety Inventory on Sleep Variables Among Young Adults (N = 359)

Variable	B	SE B	β	ΔR^2
Step 1				
SQR	−6.34	0.83	−0.37	.14

Note. Significance criterion for variable entry is $p < .05$.

TABLE A4.28
Broad Normal Sample: Stepwise Regression of the Epworth Sleepiness Scale on Sleep Variables Among Older Adults (N = 234)

Variable	B	SE B	β	ΔR^2
Step 1				
NAP	0.06	0.01	0.35	.12

Note. Significance criterion for variable entry is $p < .05$.

TABLE A4.29
Broad Normal Sample: Stepwise Regression of the Stanford Sleepiness Scale on Sleep Variables Among Older Adults (N = 234)

Variable	B	SE B	β	ΔR^2
Step 1				
NAP	0.02	0.00	0.37	.14

Note. Significance criterion for variable entry is $p < .05$.

Broad Normal Sample: Stepwise Regression of the Fatigue Severity Scale
on Sleep Variables Among Older Adults (N = 234)

Variable	B	SE B	β	ΔR^2
Step 1				
NAP	0.01	0.00	0.24	.06
Step 2				
TST	0.00	0.00	0.14	.02
Step 3				
SE	–0.04	0.01	–0.21	.04

Note. Significance criterion for variable entry is $p < .05$. Cumulative $R^2 = .11$.

TABLE A4.31
Broad Normal Sample: Stepwise Regression of the Insomnia Impact Scale
on Sleep Variables Among Older Adults (N = 234)

Variable	B	SE B	β	ΔR^2
Step 1				
NAP	0.21	0.06	0.21	.04
Step 2				
SOL	0.30	0.11	0.17	.03
Step 3				
SQR	–4.82	2.25	–0.14	.02
Step 4				
TST	0.05	0.02	0.14	.02

Note. Significance criterion for variable entry is $p < .05$. Cumulative $R^2 = .11$.

TABLE A4.32

Broad Normal Sample: Stepwise Regression of the Beck Depression Inventory on Sleep Variables Among Older Adults (N = 234)

Variable	B	SE B	β	ΔR^2
Step 1				
SQR	−2.67	0.53	−0.32	.10
Step 2				
NAP	0.06	0.01	0.24	.06
Step 3				
TST	0.01	0.01	0.15	.02

Note. Significance criterion for variable entry is $p < .05$. Cumulative $R^2 = .18$.

TABLE A4.33

Broad Normal Sample: Stepwise Regression of the State-Trait Anxiety Inventory on Sleep Variables Among Older Adults (N = 234)

Variable	B	SE B	β	ΔR^2
Step 1				
SQR	−4.49	0.77	−0.36	.13
Step 2				
NAP	0.06	0.02	0.19	.03

Note. Significance criterion for variable entry is $p < .05$. Cumulative $R^2 = .16$.

TABLE A4.34
Broad Normal Sample: Stepwise Regression of the Epworth Sleepiness Scale on Sleep Variables Among Men ($N = 294$)

Variable	B	SE B	β	ΔR^2
Step 1				
NAP	0.05	0.01	0.25	.06
Step 2				
SQR	−1.30	0.37	−0.20	.04

Note. Significance criterion for variable entry is $p < .05$. Cumulative $R^2 = .10$.

TABLE A4.35
Broad Normal Sample: Stepwise Regression of the Stanford Sleepiness Scale on Sleep Variables Among Men ($N = 294$)

Variable	B	SE B	β	ΔR^2
Step 1				
NAP	0.02	0.00	0.23	.05
Step 2				
SQR	−0.30	0.13	−0.13	.02

Note. Significance criterion for variable entry is $p < .05$. Cumulative $R^2 = .07$.

TABLE A4.36
Broad Normal Sample: Stepwise Regression of the Fatigue Severity Scale on Sleep Variables Among Men ($N = 294$)

Variable	B	SE B	β	ΔR^2
Step 1				
SQR	−0.38	0.11	−0.19	.04
Step 2				
NAP	0.01	0.00	0.18	.03
Step 3				
TST	0.00	0.00	0.14	.02

Note. Significance criterion for variable entry is $p < .05$. Cumulative $R^2 = .09$.

TABLE A4.37

Broad Normal Sample: Stepwise Regression of the Insomnia Impact Scale on Sleep Variables Among Men (N = 294)

Variable	B	SE B	β	ΔR^2
Step 1				
SQR	−7.96	2.17	−0.21	.04
Step 2				
TST	0.06	0.02	0.15	.02
Step 3				
NAP	0.14	0.06	0.13	.02

Note. Significance criterion for variable entry is $p < .05$. Cumulative $R^2 = .08$.

TABLE A4.38

Broad Normal Sample: Stepwise Regression of the Beck Depression Inventory on Sleep Variables Among Men (N = 294)

Variable	B	SE B	β	ΔR^2
Step 1				
SQR	−2.46	0.50	−0.28	.08
Step 2				
NAP	0.07	0.01	0.26	.07
Step 3				
TST	0.01	0.01	0.15	.02
Step 4				
SE	−0.11	0.05	−0.13	.01

Note. Significance criterion for variable entry is $p < .05$. Cumulative $R^2 = .18$.

TABLE A4.39
Broad Normal Sample: Stepwise Regression of the State-Trait Anxiety Inventory on Sleep Variables Among Men (N = 294)

Variable	B	SE B	β	ΔR^2
Step 1				
SQR	−5.00	0.82	−0.34	.11

Note. Significance criterion for variable entry is $p < .05$.

TABLE A4.40
Broad Normal Sample: Stepwise Regression of the Epworth Sleepiness Scale on Sleep Variables Among Women (N = 299)

Variable	B	SE B	β	ΔR^2
Step 1				
NAP	0.05	0.01	0.26	.07
Step 2				
SOL	−0.04	0.02	−0.13	.02

Note. Significance criterion for variable entry is $p < .05$. Cumulative $R^2 = .09$.

TABLE A4.41
Broad Normal Sample: Stepwise Regression of the Stanford Sleepiness Scale on Sleep Variables Among Women (N = 299)

Variable	B	SE B	β	ΔR^2
Step 1				
NAP	0.02	0.00	0.31	.10
Step 2				
SQR	−0.33	0.13	−0.14	.02

Note. Significance criterion for variable entry is $p < .05$. Cumulative $R^2 = .11$.

TABLE A4.42
Broad Normal Sample: Stepwise Regression of the Fatigue Severity Scale on Sleep Variables Among Women (N = 299)

Variable	B	SE B	β	ΔR^2
Step 1				
SQR	−0.33	0.12	−0.16	.03
Step 2				
TST	0.00	0.00	0.12	.01
Step 3				
SE	−0.02	0.01	−0.13	.01

Note. Significance criterion for variable entry is $p < .05$. Cumulative $R^2 = .05$.

TABLE A4.43
Broad Normal Sample: Stepwise Regression of the Insomnia Impact Scale on Sleep Variables Among Women (N = 299)

Variable	B	SE B	β	ΔR^2
Step 1				
SQR	−12.45	1.82	−0.37	.14
Step 2				
NWAK	−3.89	1.27	−0.17	.03
Step 3				
NAP	0.17	0.06	0.16	.02
Step 4				
TST	0.04	0.02	0.12	.01

Note. Significance criterion for variable entry is $p < .05$. Cumulative $R^2 = .20$.

TABLE A4.44
Broad Normal Sample: Stepwise Regression of the Beck Depression Inventory on Sleep Variables Among Women ($N = 299$)

Variable	B	SE B	β	ΔR^2
Step 1				
SQR	−3.45	0.60	−0.32	.10

Note. Significance criterion for variable entry is $p < .05$.

TABLE A4.45
Broad Normal Sample: Stepwise Regression of the State-Trait Anxiety Inventory on Sleep Variables Among Women ($N = 299$)

Variable	B	SE B	β	ΔR^2
Step 1				
SQR	−6.27	0.82	−0.41	.16

Note. Significance criterion for variable entry is $p < .05$.

TABLE A4.46
Narrow Normal Sample: Stepwise Regression of the Epworth Sleepiness Scale on Sleep Variables Among Young Men ($N = 132$)

Variable	B	SE B	β	ΔR^2
Step 1				
SQR	−1.67	0.59	−0.24	.06

Note. Significance criterion for variable entry is $p < .05$.

TABLE A4.47
Narrow Normal Sample: Stepwise Regression of the Stanford Sleepiness Scale on Sleep Variables Among Young Men (N = 132)

Variable	B	SE B	β	ΔR^2
Step 1				
SQR	−0.52	0.20	−0.22	.05

Note. Significance criterion for variable entry is $p < .05$.

TABLE A4.48
Narrow Normal Sample: Stepwise Regression of the Fatigue Severity Scale on Sleep Variables Among Young Men (N = 132)

Variable	B	SE B	β	ΔR^2
Step 1				
SQR	−0.55	0.16	−0.28	.08

Note. Significance criterion for variable entry is $p < .05$.

TABLE A4.49
Narrow Normal Sample: Stepwise Regression of the Insomnia Impact Scale on Sleep Variables Among Young Men (N = 132)

Variable	B	SE B	β	ΔR^2
Step 1				
SQR	−12.37	3.21	−0.32	.10
Step 2				
TST	0.09	0.04	0.20	.04
Step 3				
NAP	0.21	0.11	0.18	.03

Note. Significance criterion for variable entry is $p < .05$. Cumulative $R^2 = .17$.

TABLE A4.50
Narrow Normal Sample: Stepwise Regression of the Beck Depression Inventory on Sleep Variables Among Young Men ($N = 132$)

Variable	B	SE B	β	ΔR^2
Step 1				
WASO	0.16	0.05	0.27	.07

Note. Significance criterion for variable entry is $p < .05$.

TABLE A4.51
Narrow Normal Sample: Stepwise Regression of the State-Trait Anxiety Inventory on Sleep Variables Among Young Men ($N = 132$)

Variable	B	SE B	β	ΔR^2
Step 1				
SQR	−6.66	1.52	−0.36	.13

Note. Significance criterion for variable entry is $p < .05$.

Table A4.52
Narrow Normal Sample: Stepwise Regression of the Epworth Sleepiness Scale on Sleep Variables Among Young Women ($N = 119$)

Variable	B	SE B	β	ΔR^2
Step 1				
NAP	0.07	0.03	0.26	.07

Note. Significance criterion for variable entry is $p < .05$.

TABLE A4.53

Narrow Normal Sample: Stepwise Regression of the Stanford Sleepiness Scale on Sleep Variables Among Young Women (N = 119)

Variable	B	SE B	β	ΔR^2
Step 1				
NAP	0.03	0.01	0.33	.11

Note. Significance criterion for variable entry is $p < .05$.

TABLE A4.54

Narrow Normal Sample: Stepwise Regression of the Fatigue Severity Scale on Sleep Variables Among Young Women (N = 119)

Variable	B	SE B	β	ΔR^2
Step 1				
SQR	−0.52	0.18	−0.25	.06

Note. Significance criterion for variable entry is $p < .05$.

TABLE A4.55

Narrow Normal Sample: Stepwise Regression of the Insomnia Impact Scale on Sleep Variables Among Young Women (N = 119)

Variable	B	SE B	β	ΔR^2
Step 1				
SQR	−11.76	3.25	−0.32	.10

Note. Significance criterion for variable entry is $p < .05$.

TABLE A4.56
Narrow Normal Sample: Stepwise Regression of the Beck Depression Inventory on Sleep Variables Among Young Women (N = 119)

Variable	B	SE B	β	ΔR^2
Step 1				
SQR	−2.95	0.90	−0.29	.09

Note. Significance criterion for variable entry is $p < .05$.

TABLE A4.57
Narrow Normal Sample: Stepwise Regression of the State-Trait Anxiety Inventory on Sleep Variables Among Young Women (N = 119)

Variable	B	SE B	β	ΔR^2
Step 1				
SQR	−6.80	1.35	−0.42	.18

Note. Significance criterion for variable entry is $p < .05$.

TABLE A4.58
Narrow Normal Sample: Stepwise Regression of the Epworth Sleepiness Scale on Sleep Variables Among Old Men (N = 80)

Variable	B	SE B	β	ΔR^2
Step 1				
NAP	0.09	0.02	0.40	.16

Note. Significance criterion for variable entry is $p < .05$.

TABLE A4.59
Narrow Normal Sample: Stepwise Regression of the Stanford Sleepiness Scale on Sleep Variables Among Old Men (N = 80)

Variable	B	SE B	β	ΔR^2
Step 1				
WASO	0.04	0.02	0.23	.05

Note. Significance criterion for variable entry is $p < .05$.

TABLE A4.60
Narrow Normal Sample: Stepwise Regression of the Fatigue Severity Scale on Sleep Variables Among Old Men (N = 80)

Variable	B	SE B	β	ΔR^2
Step 1				
NAP	0.03	0.01	0.32	.10

Note. Significance criterion for variable entry is $p < .05$.

TABLE A4.61
Narrow Normal Sample: Stepwise Regression of the Beck Depression Inventory on Sleep Variables Among Old Men (N = 80)

Variable	B	SE B	β	ΔR^2
Step 1				
NAP	0.11	0.03	0.40	.16
Step 2				
SQR	−1.61	0.76	−0.22	.05
Step 3				
TST	0.01	0.01	0.20	.04

Note. Significance criterion for variable entry is $p < .05$. Cumulative $R^2 = .25$.

TABLE A4.62
Narrow Normal Sample: Stepwise Regression of the State-Trait Anxiety Inventory on Sleep Variables Among Old Men ($N = 80$)

Variable	B	SE B	β	ΔR^2
Step 1				
SQR	–3.20	1.23	–0.28	.08
Step 2				
TST	0.02	0.01	0.22	.05

Note. Significance criterion for variable entry is $p < .05$. Cumulative $R^2 = .13$.

TABLE A4.63
Narrow Normal Sample: Stepwise Regression of Epworth Sleepiness Scale on Sleep Variables Among Old Women ($N = 61$)

Variable	B	SE B	β	ΔR^2
Step 1				
NAP	0.08	0.03	0.36	.13

Note. Significance criterion for variable entry is $p < .05$.

TABLE A4.64
Narrow Normal Sample: Stepwise Regression of Stanford Sleepiness Scale on Sleep Variables Among Old Women ($N = 61$)

Variable	B	SE B	β	ΔR^2
Step 1				
NAP	0.04	0.01	0.42	.18

Note. Significance criterion for variable entry is $p < .05$.

TABLE A4.65
Narrow Normal Sample: Stepwise Regression of Fatigue Severity Scale on Sleep Variables Among Old Women (N = 61)

Variable	B	SE B	β	ΔR^2
Step 1				
NWAK	0.46	0.21	0.28	.08

Note. Significance criterion for variable entry is p < .05.

TABLE A4.66
Narrow Normal Sample: Stepwise Regression of Insomnia Impact Scale on Sleep Variables Among Old Women (N = 61)

Variable	B	SE B	β	ΔR^2
Step 1				
SOL	0.45	0.19	0.30	.09

Note. Significance criterion for variable entry is *p* < .05.

TABLE A4.67
Narrow Normal Sample: Stepwise Regression of Beck Depression Inventory on Sleep Variables Among Old Women (N = 61)

Variable	B	SE B	β	ΔR^2
Step 1				
SQR	−2.61	1.14	−0.28	.08

Note. Significance criterion for variable entry is *p* < .05.

5

An Archive of Insomnia

There are no widely accepted quantitative criteria for defining insomnia, in part explaining why prevalence for insomnia vary wildly (see chap. 2). Neither the *International Statistical Classification of Diseases and Related Health Problems, Tenth Revision* (ICD-10, World Health Organization, 1992), nor the *Diagnostic and Statistical Manual of Mental Disorders,* 4th edition (*DSM–IV,* American Psychiatric Association, 1994), nor the *International Classification of Sleep Disorders: Diagnostic and Coding Manual* (ICSD, American Sleep Disorders Association, 1990) provides adequate quantitative criteria for assigning the insomnia diagnosis (reviewed in Lichstein, Durrence, Taylor, Bush, & Riedel, 2003).

We recently derived empirically based quantitative criteria for insomnia (Lichstein et al., 2003), providing a reasoned alternative to the extant typical epidemiological practice of determining insomnia presence solely by asking individuals, do you have insomnia? We combined two approaches to establish diagnostic criteria. First, we reviewed two decades of psychology clinical trials for insomnia to determine modal practice with regard to frequency, severity, and duration criteria for insomnia. This procedure identified widely accepted frequency and duration criteria, but failed to resolve ambiguity in selecting severity criteria. Second, we applied sensitivity–specificity analyses to four common severity criteria to identify the most valid criterion. We concluded that severity of sleep onset latency (SOL) or wake time after sleep onset (WASO) of (a) ≥31 min (b) occurring ≥3 nights a week (c) for ≥6 months are the most defensible quantitative criteria for insomnia.

Poor sleep is critical to diagnosing insomnia, but it is not sufficient. We also considered evidence of daytime impairment requisite to conferring this diagnosis. This standard derives from the ICSD, which requires a report of impaired daytime functioning among insomnia criteria. The present survey included six measures of daytime impairment, but we excluded the Stanford Sleepiness Scale (SSS) from this process because we used a newly conceived trait form of this instrument. To be diagnosed as a person or people with insomnia (PWI), an individual's score had to exceed the lower boundary of impairment on at least one of the five measures. The cutoffs we used were: Epworth Sleepiness Scale (ESS) ≥ 7.4, Fatigue Severity Scale (FSS) ≥ 5.5, Insomnia Impact Scale (IIS) ≥ 125, Beck Depression Inventory (BDI) ≥ 10, or State-Trait Anxiety Inventory (STAI) ≥ 37. Justification for these cutoffs was given in Lichstein et al. (2003).

The ICSD lists two additional criteria for insomnia: (a) the self-perception of having insomnia and (b) evidence of conditioned arousal to the sleep setting. The health survey we used asked individuals to report if they had a sleep disorder. Individuals had to identify themselves as having insomnia to be counted as PWI in this survey. We did not collect any information to address criteria b, but we do not consider this a serious fault. No epidemiological survey of sleep has ever considered conditioned sleep arousal in its criteria for insomnia and, similarly, this criterion is used infrequently in other research and clinical settings.

Table 5.1 summarizes the set of criteria defining our standards for diagnosing insomnia in this survey. Individuals classified as PWI had to satisfy all criteria. These are the most specific and the most demanding criteria for identifying PWI ever used in an epidemiological study. We expect, therefore, that insomnia prevalence rates determined by this survey are conservative estimates.

Terminal insomnia or early-morning awakening was excluded from the above definition for several reasons. In our sample, only two people identified themselves as having terminal insomnia. One woman reported chronic early-morning awakenings and one man reported a recent problem with terminal insomnia. We had insufficient data to analyze this type of insomnia. Also, terminal insomnia is difficult to quantify. It refers to awakening early in the morning with the inability to return to sleep, but a quantitative standard for defining this pattern does not exist. Further, this definition presumes a reasonable bedtime. If the individual went to sleep early in the evening, early-morning awakening would be expected.

INSOMNIA PREVALENCE

We began by excluding the 10 individuals whose ethnicity was neither African American (AA) nor Caucasian (CA), as was done in chapter 4, because we later (chap. 6) compare AA and CA PWI. Applying the cri-

TABLE 5.1
Diagnostic Criteria for Insomnia Used in This Survey

Criteria	Measurement Standard
(1) Complaint of insomnia	Reported current insomnia on health survey
(2) Poor sleep	(A) SOL or WASO ≥31 min,
	(B) occurring ≥3 nights a week, and
	(C) duration ≥6 months
(3) Impaired daytime functioning on at least one of these:	
	(A) ESS ≥7.4
	(B) FSS ≥5.5
	(C) IIS ≥125
	(D) BDI ≥10
	(E) STAI ≥37

teria of Table 5.1 to the sample now numbering 762, 136 individuals qualified as PWI. This insomnia prevalence rate of 17.8% should be interpreted very cautiously. As discussed in great detail in chapter 4 (section on Generalizability of These Data: Strengths and Limitations), our sampling methods over represented older adults, and this would have an inflationary effect on the overall prevalence rate. Prevalence within age decades can be interpreted reliably.

Prevalence by Age and Gender

Table 5.2 presents prevalence data for insomnia. As is usually found in epidemiological studies, insomnia was significantly more common in women ($n = 81$) than in men ($n = 55$), $\chi^2(1, N = 136) = 4.97, p < .05$. However, the frequency distribution of PWI across decades did not show a significant differential pattern by gender, $\chi^2(6, N = 136) = 3.56, ns$. Gender not considered, the prevalence of insomnia did rise with advancing age, $\chi^2(6, N = 136) = 20.27, p < .01$.

TABLE 5.2
Prevalence of Insomnia

Age	Frequency		Prevalence[a]	
	M	W	M	W
20–29	3	6	.06 (50)	.12 (52)
30–39	11	8	.22 (51)	.12 (68)
40–49	6	10	.11 (54)	.20 (51)
50–59	6	12	.10 (58)	.21 (58)
60–69	5	9	.09 (54)	.17 (52)
70–79	12	15	.23 (53)	.26 (58)
80–89+	12	21	.23 (52)	.41 (51)
Total	55	81	.15 (372)	.21 (390)

Note. M = men and W = women.
[a]Prevalence by decade. The insomnia frequency in each decade is affected by the number of men and women present in the sample in that decade, and in most decades this was not exactly even. Insomnia frequency for each gender is referenced to the total number of AA and CA men or women in each decade. The total number of men and women is given in parentheses. These counts were taken from Appendix Tables A4.15 to A4.21.

The 55 men and 81 women accounted for 40% and 60% of the PWI. Except for decade 30, this ratio was fairly consistent.

The last two columns of Table 5.2 present insomnia prevalence data by gender and decade referenced to the actual count of men and women present in those cells. It is now apparent that the overall insomnia rate of 17.8% given earlier is highly unrepresentative of most age × gender subgroups. Insomnia prevalence ranges from 6% (men, decade 20) to 41% (women, decade 80).

Decade 30 is aberrant for men. It is the only decade in which insomnia prevalence in men is greater than women, and during the middle years, it is the only decade in which male insomnia prevalence strays substantially from about 10%.

Insomnia prevalence increases in decades 70 and 80. The change is dramatic in both these decades for men and in decade 80 for women. Insomnia prevalence for men in these two decades more than doubles their rate in every other decade, except for decade 30. Decade 70 for women reveals an increase in insomnia, but it is no more than a moderate increase over the previous three decades. Insomnia in women during decade 80 is a huge outlier compared to any other age × gender cell.

The prevalence of insomnia among women about doubles that of men in decades 20, 40, 50, 60, and 80. Overall, insomnia prevalence among women (21%) is 40% higher than that among men (15%).

Comparing our data to the extant epidemiological literature (see chap. 2), we employed more conservative criteria and observed a narrower range of prevalence. According to Table 2.1, insomnia prevalence ranges from 1.6% to 67.5%. Our range in cells was 6 to 41%. Considering the middle years only (decades 30, 40, 50, and 60) in the present sample, insomnia prevalence for men was 13% (28/217) and for women 17% (39/229). In the later years (decades 70 and 80), this rises to 23% in men (24/105) or a 77% rise and 33% in women (36/109) or a 94% rise.

Population Prevalence

We now engage in an extrapolation exercise to correct for our sampling procedure by weighting our insomnia prevalence data by the distribution of age and gender in the population to yield a population estimate of insomnia. Although this approach does not absolutely erase the interpretive constraints imposed by our sampling methods discussed earlier in this chapter and in chapter 4, it is an unbiased estimating procedure, and likely produces a value closely approximating population prevalence. We believe producing a point prevalence for insomnia is an important achievement, and this is the only time in this book that we will contrive a population point estimate.

Table 5.3 presents the data we used for these calculations. Columns 1, 2, and 3 were copied from the year 2000 census data (U.S. Census Bureau, 2000). Note that these data were originally presented in 5-year increments, and we merged age groups to produce 10-year intervals matching our data set. We computed columns 4 and 5 to obtain the population proportion per age group based on adults only, because children do not contribute to the population of PWI. Columns 6 and 7 present insomnia prevalence by gender and age in our sample (taken from Table 5.2). Columns 8 and 9 are the product of columns 4 × 6 and 5 × 7, respectively, producing the weighted prevalence per age group by gender. The sum of columns 8 and 9 is the insomnia prevalence in the United States by gender.

TABLE 5.3
Weighted Prevalence Estimate of Insomnia

1	2	3	4	5	6	7	8	9
Age groups	Women[a]	Men[a]	Proportion of adult women	Proportion of adult men	Percent insomnia women[b]	Percent insomnia men[b]	Proportion of women × Percent insomnia	Proportion of men × Percent insomnia
20 to 29	18,017	18,300	0.175	0.193	11.5	6.0	2.0	1.2
30 to 39	20,977	20,630	0.204	0.218	11.8	21.6	2.4	4.7
40 to 49	21,675	21,152	0.211	0.223	19.6	11.1	4.1	2.5
50 to 59	16,041	15,038	0.156	0.159	20.7	10.3	3.2	1.6
60 to 69	10,754	9,417	0.105	0.099	17.3	9.3	1.8	0.9
70 to 79	9,188	6,995	0.089	0.074	25.9	22.6	2.3	1.7
80 to 89	4,905	2,796	0.048	0.030	41.3	22.5	2.0	0.7
90 to 99	1,157	409	0.011	0.004	40.0	33.3	0.4	0.1
100 +	56	12	0.001	0.000	0	0	0	0
Total	102,771	94,749	1.0	1.0	20.8%	14.8%	18.2%	13.4%

[a]Population in thousands.
[b]Table 5.2, from which the data in columns 6 and 7 are derived, did not separate the 80–89 and 90–99 age groups. Those data are separated in the present table.

The adult population of the United States is 197,520,000 (sum columns 2 and 3, Table 5.3). The gender weights are women = 52.03% and men = 47.97%. Multiplying the gender weights by the gender prevalence estimates (sum columns 8 and 9) and summing these two products, we obtain 15.9%, the point prevalence of insomnia in the United States. Compare this to the unweighted insomnia prevalence in our sample, 17.8%. Multiplying the adult population of the United States by 15.9% produces a rounded estimate of 31.4 million PWI in the United States.

SLEEP BY AGE AND GENDER

We used the same multivariate analysis of variance (MANOVA) model applied with normal samples in chapter 4 with one exception. The available number of PWI, 136, is not adequate to conduct a three-way analysis. With 7 levels of age, 2 gender, and 2 ethnicity, the 28 cells would average 5 individuals each, providing insufficient power to permit reasonable hypothesis testing. Therefore, we dropped the ethnicity factor for the present and focus on AA in the next chapter.

We performed a two-factor MANOVA, 7 age decades × 2 gender, for seven sleep measures, SOL, number of awakenings during the night (NWAK), WASO, total sleep time (TST), sleep efficiency percent (SE), sleep quality rating (SQR), and time spent napping (NAP). Neither the main effect for age, Wilks' $\Lambda = 0.62$, $F(42, 547) = 1.39$, $p = .06$, nor the main effect for gender, Wilks' $\Lambda = 0.94$, $F(7, 116) = 1.05$, $p = .40$, nor their interaction, Wilks' $\Lambda = 0.76$, $F(42, 547) = 0.79$, $p = .82$, attained significance. These results do not justify breaking down the sleep data by cells. Table 5.4 presents means (and SDs) for sleep measures collapsed across age and gender.

Table 5.4 reveals unambiguous sleep disturbance in this sample. SOL, WASO, and SE reflect very poor sleep. TST is at 6.4 h of sleep, well below the customary prescription of 7.5 h. The NAP value is remarkably high. PWI are not usually known for napping. In contrast to the other sleep measures, NWAK and SQR are not particularly poor. Duration of insomnia is another index of severity. Our sample of PWI reported having insomnia an average of 9.4 years ($SD = 11.5$), with a range from 6 months to 70 years. We later compare sleep in normals and PWI.

The MANOVA results for gender and the age × gender interaction reported earlier were unambiguous. We feel comfortable asserting that there is no reliable difference in the sleep of men and women with insomnia.

The near significant findings for the age factor do not so neatly erase ambiguity. On the average, we had fewer than 20 participants per age

TABLE 5.4
Mean and SD for Sleep Measures in PWI

Variable	M	SD
SOL	42.3	24.8
NWAK	2.2	1.2
WASO	53.8	41.0
TST	384.0	72.7
SE	75.5	9.5
SQR	2.9	0.6
NAP	24.4	24.8

group for this analysis, and this may have resulted in a low-power test. Inspection of the univariate tests of the seven sleep measures, however, does not support the view that the MANOVA concealed significant relationships. Only one variable, WASO, produced a significant univariate effect for age. But low power may have elevated Type II error in the univariate tests as well.

We next present the sleep data by age graphically so that the reader can inspect age trends. Because these data were nonsignificant, we forgo the more specific tabular presentation of means.

As might be expected when the probability level is near significant, some of the sleep measures show age trends. Most notably, there is substantial deterioration in SOL during decade 80 (Fig. 5.1), in NWAK during decades 60, 70, and 80 (Fig. 5.2), in WASO during decades 70 and 80 (Fig. 5.3), in SE during decades 70 and 80 (Fig. 5.5), and in NAP during decade 80 (Fig. 5.7). TST (Fig. 5.4) and SQR (Fig. 5.6) did not exhibit strong age effects.

When age-related sleep deterioration did occur, it was most likely to occur in decades 70 and 80. To achieve a more powerful statistical test of age-related changes in sleep among PWI, we collapsed decades 20 to 60 and 70 to 80 and performed a multivariate t-test. This analysis provides a contrasting view. We now observe a significant age effect, Wilks' $\Lambda = 0.80$, $F(7, 128) = 4.48$, $p < .01$. As suggested by Figs. 5.2, 5.3, and 5.5, univariate analyses revealed that the NWAK, WASO, and SE are significantly worse in older adults than younger adults (see Table 5.5). The re-

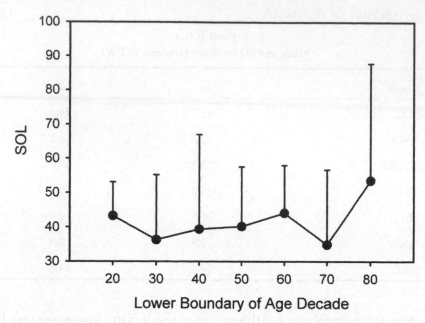

FIG. 5.1. Mean (and *SD* bar) sleep onset latency (minutes) by decade in people with insomnia.

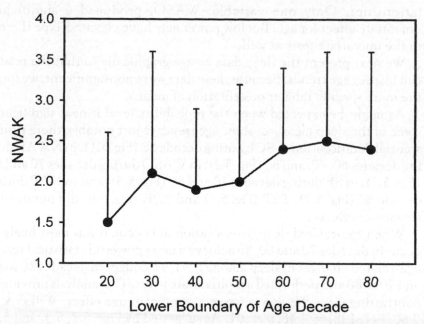

FIG. 5.2. Mean (and *SD* bar) number of awakenings by decade in people with insomnia.

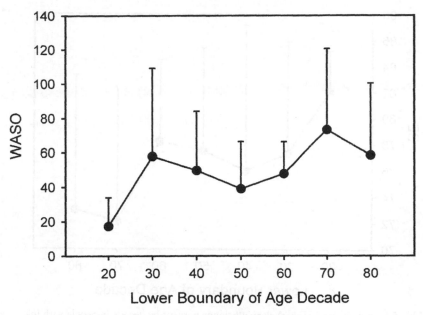

FIG. 5.3. Mean (and SD bar) wake time after sleep onset (minutes) by decade in people with insomnia.

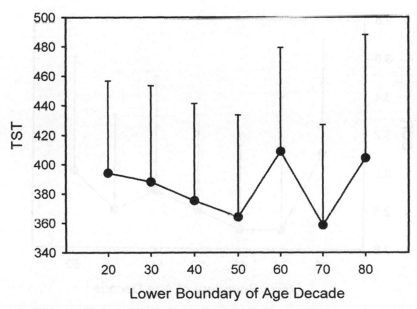

FIG. 5.4. Mean (and SD bar) total sleep time (minutes) by decade in people with insomnia.

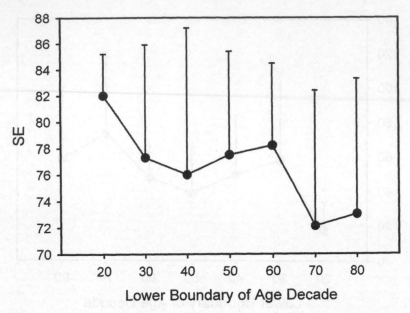

FIG. 5.5.   Mean (and *SD* bar) sleep efficiency percent by decade in people with insomnia.

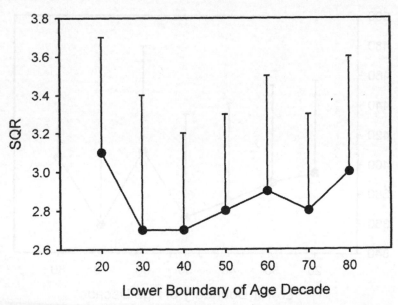

FIG. 5.6.   Mean (and *SD* bar) sleep quality rating by decade in people with insomnia.

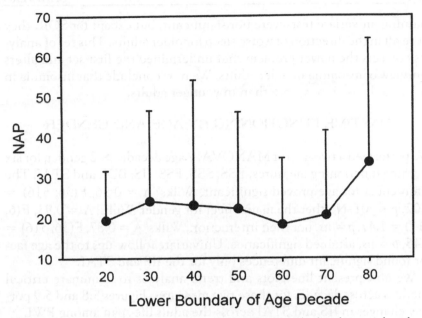

FIG. 5.7.   Mean (and SD bar) time spent napping (minutes) by decade in people with insomnia.

TABLE 5.5
Mean and SD Comparing Sleep Measures in Young and Older PWI

Variable	Younger Adults Ages 20–69		Older Adults Ages 70–89+	
	M	SD	M	SD
SOL	40.1	18.9	45.1	30.6
NWAK*	2.0	1.2	2.5	1.1
WASO**	45.0	35.8	65.0	44.7
TST	384.2	67.1	383.8	79.8
SE**	77.8	8.2	72.6	10.2
SQR	2.8	0.6	2.9	0.6
NAP	21.8	22.5	27.7	27.2

*$p < .05$. **$p < .01$.

maining univariate tests were nonsignificant, but except for SQR, they were all in the direction of worse sleep for older adults. This set of analyses corrects the power problem that undermined the first set and alters our view of insomnia in older adults. We now conclude that insomnia in older adults is more severe than in younger adults.

DAYTIME FUNCTIONING BY AGE AND GENDER

We performed a two-factor MANOVA, 7 age decades × 2 gender, for six daytime functioning measures, ESS, SSS, FSS, IIS, BDI, and STAI. The main effect for age proved significant, Wilks' Λ = 0.56, $F(36, 516)$ = 2.02, p < .01. Neither the main effect for gender, Wilks' Λ = 0.93, $F(6, 117)$ = 1.47, p = ns, nor their interaction, Wilks' Λ = 0.87, $F(36, 516)$ = 0.45, p = ns, attained significance. Univariate follow-ups to the age factor found significant differences only for the IIS and STAI.

We now present line plots and trend analyses to illuminate critical changes across decades for these two measures. Figures 5.8 and 5.9 portray changes in IIS and STAI across the adult life span among PWI.

The two measures exhibit a similar pattern. Both had significant cubic trends characterized by relatively high values in the early adult years, im-

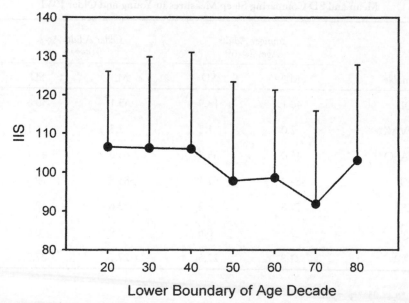

FIG. 5.8.   Mean (and SD bar) Insomnia Impact Scale by decade in people with insomnia.

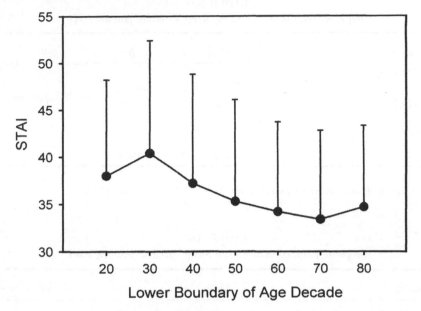

FIG. 5.9.   Mean (and *SD* bar) State Trait Anxiety Inventory by decade in people with insomnia.

proving in the middle years, and reversing the improvement trend in decade 80. At the least, we can conclude that in these two measures (and the other nonsignificant daytime measures), older PWI do not suffer greater daytime impairment than younger PWI.

A different view of the association between sleep and daytime functioning can be gained by adopting the analytic approach of chapter 4. We conducted a series of stepwise multiple regression analyses regressing each of the six daytime functioning instruments on the set of seven sleep measures collapsing across age and gender.

Two sleep variables accounted for 17% of the variance in ESS (Table 5.6). Increased NAP and shorter SOL were associated with greater daytime sleepiness as measured by the ESS.

With our second measure of daytime sleepiness, SSS, increased NAP and decreased TST (explaining 12% of variance) were associated with higher SSS scores (Table 5.7).

The regression of FSS on sleep proved nonsignificant. SQR ratings were associated with all three remaining daytime variables (Tables 5.8, 5.9, and 5.10). For IIS, lower SQR and longer SOL (11% variance combined) were related to greater insomnia impact; for BDI, lower SQR and

TABLE 5.6
Stepwise Regression of ESS on Sleep Variables Among PWI

Variable	B	SE B	β	ΔR^2
Step 1				
NAP	0.06	0.02	0.34	.12
Step 2				
SOL	−0.04	0.02	−0.23	.05

Note. Significance criterion for variable entry is $p < .05$. Cumulative $R^2 = .17$.

TABLE 5.7
Stepwise Regression of SSS on Sleep Variables Among PWI

Variable	B	SE B	β	ΔR^2
Step 1				
NAP	0.02	0.01	0.30	.09
Step 2				
TST	−0.004	0.00	−0.18	.03

Note. Significance criterion for variable entry is $p < .05$. Cumulative $R^2 = .12$.

TABLE 5.8
Stepwise Regression of IIS on Sleep Variables Among PWI

Variable	B	SE B	β	ΔR^2
Step 1				
SQR	−10.01	3.66	−0.23	.05
Step 2				
SOL	0.24	0.08	0.24	.06

Note. Significance criterion for variable entry is $p < .05$. Cumulative $R^2 = .11$.

TABLE 5.9
Stepwise Regression of BDI on Sleep Variables Among PWI

Variable	B	SE B	β	ΔR^2
Step 1				
SQR	–4.10	1.31	–0.26	.07
Step 2				
NAP	0.07	0.03	0.19	.04

Note. Significance criterion for variable entry is $p < .05$. Cumulative $R^2 = .11$.

TABLE 5.10
Stepwise Regression of STAI on Sleep Variables Among PWI

Variable	B	SE B	β	ΔR^2
Step 1				
SQR	–5.03	1.66	–0.25	.06

Note. Significance criterion for variable entry is $p < .05$. Cumulative $R^2 = .06$.

increased NAP (11% variance combined) were related to increased depression; and for STAI, lower SQR scores alone (6% variance) were associated with greater anxiety.

In summary, the association between sleep and daytime functioning was not particularly strong among our PWI. Explained variance peaked at 17%. SQR and NAP were the sleep characteristics most indicative of daytime impairment.

INSOMNIA TYPES

Prevalence of Types

The use of quantitative criteria to define insomnia creates the opportunity to also define insomnia types. We derived four types of insomnia: onset, maintenance, mixed, and combined. Their definitions are given in Table 5.11.

TABLE 5.11
Diagnostic Criteria for Insomnia Types

Type	Definition
Onset	Satisfies quantitative criteria for onset insomnia only (SOL ≥31 min, ≥3 nights a week)
Maintenance	Satisfies quantitative criteria for maintenance insomnia only (WASO ≥31 min, ≥3 nights a week)
Mixed	Does not separately satisfy quantitative criteria for onset or maintenance insomnia, but has at least 3 insomnia nights a week (1 or 2 nights of SOL ≥31 min, and 1 or 2 nights of WASO ≥31 min)
Combined	Separately satisfies quantitative criteria for both onset and maintenance insomnia (SOL ≥31 min, ≥3 nights a week, and WASO ≥31 min, ≥3 nights a week)

Our 136 PWI were distributed among these four types as follows: 31 people had onset insomnia (22.8%), 43 maintenance (31.6%), 23 mixed (16.9%), and 39 combined (28.7%). There was no significant difference in frequency among these four categories, $\chi^2(3, N = 136) = 6.94, ns$.

The categories can be reconfigured to reflect shared components. Sleep onset problems were present in the 93 people diagnosed as onset, mixed, or combined insomnia. Thus, 68% of our insomnia sample (93/136) experienced sleep onset problems. Sleep maintenance problems were present in the 105 people diagnosed as maintenance, mixed, or combined insomnia. Thus, 77% of our insomnia sample (105/136) experienced maintenance problems. Overall, we conclude that sleep disturbances of both a sleep onset and sleep maintenance nature are widely distributed among PWI.

We explored the distribution of insomnia types across age. The common wisdom holds that onset insomnia predominates among younger people and maintenance insomnia among older people. Contrary to this expectation, the chi-square test of independence evaluating the distribution of types across decades was nonsignificant, $\chi^2(18, N = 136) = 23.85, ns$.

Figure 5.10 portrays the proportional distribution of insomnia types within decades. These data yield numerous instructive conclusions.

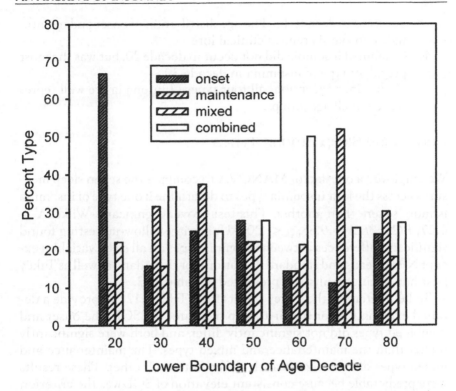

FIG. 5.10. The distribution of insomnia types by age. Bars represent proportional distribution within decades.

1. Onset insomnia, which is reputed to predominate in the early adult and middle years, was dominant in decade 20 and none other. It accounted for 67% of insomnia in this decade.
2. Maintenance insomnia, which is reputed to predominate in the later years, stood out in decade 70 and none other. It accounted for 52% of insomnia in this decade.
3. Although the strongest prevalence of onset and maintenance insomnia was in the predicted age ranges, neighboring age decades did not confirm this pattern. For example, onset insomnia was weakly represented in decade 30, and decade 80 witnessed little difference between onset (24%) and maintenance (30%) insomnia. Further, combined insomnia, defined by clinically significant onset and maintenance insomnia, was dominant (50%) in decade 60, and the second highest level of maintenance insomnia (38%)

occurred in decade 40. The age distribution of onset and maintenance insomnia refutes clinical lore.

4. Combined insomnia did not occur in decade 20, but was the most
   prevalent type of insomnia in decade 30.
5. With minor exception, all four types of insomnia are well represented in all age groups.

Comparing Sleep Among Types

We employed a one-factor MANOVA to compare the seven sleep measures across the four insomnia types to determine if one type of insomnia
is more severe than another. This test proved significant, Wilks' Λ =
0.27, $F(21, 362) = 9.88$, $p < .001$. Univariate follow-up testing found
significant differences between insomnia types on all sleep variables except NAP. Means and standard deviations for these data, as well as Tukey
post hoc testing results, are presented in Table 5.12.

To help interpret the Tukey results from Table 5.12, we provide a detailed explanation for the first sleep measure. On SOL, the onset and
combined types did not significantly differ, and both were significantly
higher than the maintenance and mixed types. The maintenance and
mixed types did not significantly differ from each other. These results
were predictable because consistent elevation of SOL was the criterion
for defining onset and combined types.

NWAK was not a diagnostic criterion, and the pattern of results for
this measure were more complex. To highlight these findings, the combined type reported the highest number of awakenings, and this was significantly greater than two of the groups, mixed and onset. The
maintenance type did not significantly differ from the combined type.

For WASO, the maintenance and combined types did not differ and
both were significantly greater than the remaining two. These results
were also constrained by diagnostic criteria.

The onset group had the best TST and the maintenance and combined groups the worst. SE showed a similar pattern. The main difference here was that the combined type was significantly worse than the
maintenance type. With SQR, maintenance and combined groups again
scored the poorest compared to onset and mixed groups.

There are clear differences in severity between insomnia types, but
the pattern is not completely consistent across sleep measures. The
Tukey results generally indicate mixed and onset types are less severe
than maintenance and combined.

TABLE 5.12
Mean and SD Comparing Sleep Measures in Insomnia Types

Variable	Onset		Maintenance		Mixed		Combined		Differences Between Types[a]
	M	SD	M	SD	M	SD	M	SD	
SOL	54.9	15.5	22.2	13.8	31.2	8.9	61.1	26.6	O = C > MA = MI
NWAK	1.3	0.9	2.6	1.1	1.9	0.9	2.8	1.2	C > MI = O; C = MA; MA = MI; MA > O
WASO	17.9	14.2	76.4	45.4	30.6	9.4	71.3	34.9	MA = C > MI = O
TST	419.3	82.5	374.6	69.1	398.1	43.5	358.1	71.4	O > MA = C; O = MI; MI = MA = C
SE	81.0	5.9	74.8	10.3	81.9	3.4	68.2	8.0	O = MI > MA > C
SQR	3.2	0.6	2.7	0.5	3.1	0.5	2.6	0.5	O = MI > MA = C
NAP	21.2	19.5	22.8	22.0	19.2	17.4	31.9	33.0	

[a]O = onset insomnia, MA = maintenance insomnia, MI = mixed insomnia, and C = combined insomnia. In summarizing the results of Tukey post hoc testing, = signifies no significant difference and > signifies the presence and direction of significant differences.

To further clarify these relationships, we conducted pairwise MANOVAs comparing the four types on the set of sleep measures with Bonferroni corrected Type I error rates, that is, $.05/6 = .008\ \alpha$. All six comparisons were significant, and the accompanying pairwise univariate results clarified the ordering of severity. The unambiguous sequence of severity from mildest to most severe is onset, mixed, maintenance, and combined.

Comparing Daytime Functioning Among Types

A MANOVA compared the four insomnia types on the set of daytime functioning measures, ESS, SSS, FSS, IIS, BDI, and STAI, and this proved nonsignificant, Wilks' $\Lambda = 0.81$, $F(18, 360) = 1.51$, $p = .08$. We continued to explore this area because the results were near significant, but our efforts proved fruitless. As with the multivariate follow-up on the sleep measures, we conducted pairwise MANOVAs on the set of daytime functioning measures. Not one of the tests proved significant, even at the .05 α level. Lastly, we attempted to maximize power by combining the two less severe groups, onset and mixed, and contrasting them with the combination of the two most severe groups, maintenance and combined. This too proved nonsignificant. We therefore feel confident in concluding that, unlike gradation in sleep severity between insomnia types, daytime functioning does not vary with type.

COMPARING PWI AND PEOPLE
NOT HAVING INSOMNIA (PNI)

Quantitative criteria identified 136 PWI, and these were compared to the narrow normal sample defined in chapter 4. We chose this particular normal sample from among the three identified in chapter 4 because it captures the best sleep reasonably possible for PWI. By comparing the experience of PWI to a group representing goal sleep, we can estimate how much change is needed among PWI for them to attain *desired, normal* status.

Demographics

We began by comparing the two groups on a number of demographic variables. As shown in Table 5.13, *t*-tests revealed that PWI are significantly older and less educated (based on highest household education) than PNI. PWI list a significantly greater number of medical problems

TABLE 5.13
Mean and SD Comparing Demographics in PWI and PNI

Variable	PWI		PNI	
	M	SD	M	SD
Age***	60.5	20.0	50.6	19.0
Education***	13.4	2.8	14.6	2.8
BMI	27.1	6.3	26.2	5.1
Illness count***	2.2	1.6	0.8	1.1
Medication count***	3.4	2.8	1.7	1.9
Alcohol (week)	1.9	4.9	2.7	5.2
Cigarettes (day)	4.2	10.2	4.1	9.5
Caffeine (day)	2.3	2.8	2.3	2.4

***$p < .001$.

and report taking more medications than PNI. There was no significant difference between the two groups on body mass index (BMI), number of alcoholic drinks per week, number of cigarettes per day, or number of caffeinated beverages per day. We can offer two brief observations on these findings. First, it is not surprising that medical illness indicators are higher in PWI, because past research has reported similar findings (Riedel & Lichstein, 2000), and medical problems are a common cause of insomnia (Lichstein, 2000). Second, we were relieved to learn that PWI were not consuming elevated levels of caffeine, but, unfortunately, nor were they consuming less than PNI. If someone is dissatisfied with their sleep, restricting caffeine is the easiest, cheapest, and safest intervention, and, for some individuals, a highly effective one as well.

We also applied chi-square tests to three other demographics. There was no significant difference in the distribution of ethnicity among PWI and PNI, $\chi^2(1, N = 528) = 1.14$, ns. Women were overrepresented among PWI (59.6% of sample) compared to PNI (45.9% of sample), $\chi^2(1, N = 528) = 7.52, p < .01$. As with medical complaints, more PWI reported mental health disorders (13.2% of sample) than did PNI (3.8% of sample), $\chi^2(1, N = 528) = 15.26, p < .001$.

Sleep

We performed a MANOVA comparing PWI and PNI on the set of sleep variables. Based on participant selection criteria, differences between these groups were designed. Of interest is the magnitude of the difference. As expected, the sleep measures were significantly different between the groups, Wilks' $\Lambda = 0.37$, $F(7, 520) = 124.77$, $p < .001$. Mean sleep in these two groups is given in Table 5.14. Univariate t-tests comparing the groups found a significant difference on every sleep variable, all $p < .001$. And, of course, in every case PWI slept worse than PNI.

Table 5.14 also presents the difference between the means of the groups on each variable. Dividing the difference by the PWI mean and multiplying by 100 produces the percent change needed by the average PWI to attain the PNI mean. Thus, on the average, PWI would have to decrease SOL 66.2% to match the PNI mean SOL. PWI would have to decrease NWAK 45.5%, decrease WASO 79.7%, increase TST 12.8%, increase SE 20.8%, increase SQR 27.6%, and decrease NAP 45.9%. SOL, WASO, and SE are particularly daunting.

TABLE 5.14

Mean and SD Comparing Sleep Measures in PWI and PNI

Variable	PWI		PNI		M Difference
	M	SD	M	SD	
SOL	42.3	24.8	14.3	8.7	28.0
NWAK	2.2	1.2	1.2	0.9	1.0
WASO	53.8	41.0	10.9	9.1	42.9
TST	384.0	72.7	433.2	58.7	49.2
SE	75.5	9.5	91.2	4.3	15.7
SQR	2.9	0.6	3.7	0.6	0.8
NAP	24.4	24.8	13.2	17.2	11.2

Note. All comparisons are significant at $p < .001$.

Daytime Functioning

The same analytic approach yielded parallel findings for daytime functioning. The MANOVA was significant, Wilks' $\Lambda = 0.72$, $F(6, 521) = 34.29$, $p < .001$. Mean daytime functioning in these two groups is given in Table 5.15. Univariate t-tests comparing the groups found a significant difference on every variable, all $p < .001$. And in every case PWI reported greater daytime impairment than PNI.

Using the mean difference scores from Table 5.15, we can estimate percent change needed for the PWI group to match the PNI group mean. ESS among PWI would have to decrease on average 17.3% to attain the ESS level of PNI. Similarly, SSS would have to decrease 29.7%, FSS decrease 27.3%, IIS decrease 17.6%, BDI decrease 59.0%, and STAI decrease 23.9%.

It is important to recognize although PWI report greater daytime impairment than PNI, the mean level of impairment for PWI on these measures is usually subclinical. Clearly, PWI scores on the FSS (Lichstein, Means, Noe, & Aguillard, 1997), the IIS (Hoelscher, Ware, & Bond, 1993), and the BDI (Beck & Steer, 1987) do not exceed the mild range. The ESS for PWI are higher than anticipated, but so too are the scores

TABLE 5.15
Mean and SD Comparing Daytime Functioning Measures in PWI and PNI

| Variable | PWI | | PNI | | |
	M	SD	M	SD	M Difference
ESS	9.8	4.5	8.1	4.0	1.7
SSS	3.7	1.5	2.6	1.5	1.1
FSS	4.4	1.3	3.2	1.2	1.2
IIS	114.7	25.0	94.5	21.8	20.2
BDI	13.9	9.0	5.7	5.3	8.2
STAI	43.5	11.4	33.1	9.3	10.4

Note. All comparisons are significant at $p < .001$.

for PNI on this measure (Johns & Hocking, 1997). The ESS has not been carefully normed. The STAI is the only measure that appears to be in the clinically significant range for PWI and is in the normal range for PNI (Spielberger, Gorsuch, Lushene, Vagg, & Jacobs, 1983).

6

An Archive of the Sleep of African Americans

The disadvantaged health experience of African Americans (AA) has been carefully documented (Livingston, 1994). Compared to Caucasians (CA), AA have a higher prevalence of stroke, hypertension, glaucoma, and kidney disease. Aside from frequency, illness severity, as indicated by associated mortality, is often higher in AA than CA as well. The death rate from infant mortality, heart disease, cirrhosis, diabetes, asthma, and stroke is 50% to 150% greater in AA than CA. AA also experience substantially higher death rate for cancer and death by homicide.

At the same time that AA experience more frequent and more severe illness, economic and sociological barriers contribute to their underutilization and diminished quality of health care services (Davis & Rowland, 1983; Jones & Rene, 1994; Kahn et al., 1994; Murrell, Smith, Gill, & Oxley, 1996; Snowden, 2001). Not surprisingly, as of 1995, AA life expectancy is 6 (women) to 8 (men) years less than that of CA (Macera, Armstead, & Anderson, 2001). The health and health care for AA are clearly compromised.

Many of the barriers to health care utilization among AA also contribute to discouraging AA participation in health research. It is well documented that AA are underrepresented in health research, and reasons for this include distrust of the medical establishment, anticipation of discrepant quality of care, constricted health knowledge, and higher costs associated with recruiting AA (Corbie-Smith, Thomas, & St. George, 2002; Shavers-Hornaday, Lynch, Burmeister, & Torner, 1997). Research on the sleep of AA has not been spared such obstacles. Sleep in AA, as a subset of health, has received even less attention than many other areas.

We (Durrence & Lichstein, 2003) recently reviewed the empirical literature on the sleep of AA, and the gaps in information are more prominent than the accumulated knowledge. Based on a relatively small number of studies, the following conclusions comparing the sleep of AA and CA appear justified, at least on a preliminary basis:

1. Sleep is lighter in AA.
2. AA sleep longer than CA.
3. AA nap more than CA.
4. Among older adults, differences between AA and CA sleep diminish.
5. Insomnia prevalence and insomnia severity is worse in AA.
6. Sleep apnea is more prevalent in AA.
7. There are no data on treating sleep disorders in AA.

The present data set, given its size and breadth, represents the most thorough accounting of the sleep of AA to date.

METHODS OF STATISTICAL ANALYSIS

We observe the general strategies laid out in chapter 4. This chapter also raises new analytic challenges in performing numerous comparisons between AA and CA. Because these two groups may differ on a number of demographic characteristics that may also influence sleep, the question of using covariates in analyses (ANCOVA) naturally arises. Our perspective on ANCOVA and its applicability to these data follows.

Covariates are most commonly used under two circumstances (Maxwell & Delaney, 1990, chap. 9; Winer, 1971, chap. 10): (1) to reduce error variance when a variable of no direct interest of study is correlated with the outcome measure and (2) to equate groups on such variables.

In both cases, *nuisance* variables are identified and their incorporation into the statistical model will alter the treatment effect and the power of the analysis. In the first case, the effect is almost always to increase power.

In the second case, the goal is to repair confounded designs, the mechanism is to conduct analyses on adjusted means that equate groups on the covariate, and the effect on power will vary. Further, the interpretation of the outcome may be cloudy because the adjusted means may be highly divergent from the raw means (Huitema, 1980, chap. 7; Maxwell & Delaney, 1990, chap. 9)

For each sample subset that follows, broad normal sample, narrow normal sample, and people with insomnia (PWI), we engaged the following procedure. To identify good covariates, we began by selecting sleep efficiency percent (SE) as a representative sleep measure and correlated it with a list of plausible demographics that might be associated with sleep: (a) gender, (b) age, (c) highest education level in the household (as a proxy for socioeconomic status), (d) body mass index (BMI, the ratio of metric weight/height^2), (e) number of illnesses currently reported, (f) number of medications currently taken, (g) number of caffeinated drinks per day, (h) number of cigarettes smoked per day, and (i) number of alcoholic drinks per week. Significant correlations > .2, that is, accounting for at least 4% of explained variance (r^2), will be recruited as covariates.

Second, we also explored differences between AA and CA on these potential covariates. Significant group mean differences having at least a moderate effect size (d; Cohen, 1987) were also recruited as covariates. Given our large sample size, small differences may prove to be statistically significant, but such contrasts are not necessarily of meaningful magnitude. For this judgment we rely on Cohen's general guideline that effect sizes may be small ($d = 0.2$), medium ($d = 0.5$), or large ($d = 0.8$). The signs of d were contrived so that positive d reflects an advantage to AA.

For each analysis, we report the ANOVA in detail and if the ANCOVA significantly changes the results, we will report its findings as well. This approach permits us to examine the raw and adjusted means, and subsequently to arrive at a more clear understanding of the analyses.

AA SLEEP IN THE BROAD NORMAL SAMPLE

The broad normal sample comprises 593 people, 178 AA (79 men and 99 women) and 415 CA (215 men and 200 women). Chapter 4 found a main effect for ethnicity and an age × ethnicity interaction on the set of sleep measures. We now explore this interaction.

Covariates

We began by attempting to identify potent covariates from among the set of plausible variables already identified. Age was excluded from this list because it is being retained as a factor. Table 6.1 shows that all but one of the variables were significantly related to SE, although the correlations were modest and the explained variance, r^2, trivial.

We further pursued identifying useful covariates by conducting t-tests comparing the two ethnic groups on each of these variables excepting for the nominal variable gender. These results are given in Table 6.2.

TABLE 6.1
Pearson Correlation Between Sleep Efficiency Percent and Plausibly
Related Demographics in the Broad Normal Sample

Demographic	n^a	r	r^2
Gender[b]	593	$-.14**$	.02
Education	504	$.17***$	.03
BMI	589	$-.14***$	.02
Illness count	593	$-.14**$	.02
Medication count	593	$-.12**$	.01
Caffeine	588	$.09*$	.01
Cigarettes	590	$.10*$	.01
Alcohol	591	$.03$	0

[a]Variations in n are due to missing data.
[b]By our coding scheme, the negative correlation reflects better sleep for men. $*p < .05$. $**p <$ .01. $***p < .001$.

TABLE 6.2
Comparison of AA and CA on Potential Covariates
in the Broad Normal Sample

	AA		CA		
Variable	M	SD	M	SD	d^a
Education***	13.2	3.1	15.0	2.6	−0.66
BMI***	28.0	6.1	25.7	4.8	−0.44
Illness count	0.9	1.1	1.0	1.2	
Medication count***	1.4	2.0	2.1	2.1	0.32
Caffeine***	1.4	1.5	2.6	2.5	0.51
Cigarettes	2.7	7.7	4.1	9.7	
Alcohol***	1.5	3.2	3.1	6.2	0.28

[a]Positive signs reflect favorably on AA and negative signs reflect favorably on CA. $***p < .001$.

Significant differences were found for all but two of the variables, illness count and cigarette consumption. The direction of difference on
the means revealed an advantage to AA on five of seven variables. For
example, on average, AA reported fewer medications, consumed less
caffeine, and consumed less alcohol. No effect size was large (computed
only for significant variables), and only two were medium, education
level and caffeine. The comparison of gender distribution by ethnic
group proved nonsignificant, $\chi^2(1, N = 593) = 2.75, ns.$

These analyses steer us to use gender, education, BMI, illness count,
medication count, and caffeine as covariates. The rationale for this decision derives from the guidelines established above for covariate selection.
We had hoped to use an $r > .2$ cutoff for one criterion, but none of the rs
were this strong. We therefore reconsidered this criterion and selected the
five variables whose rs clustered in the teens (Table 6.1). Using the effect
size criterion (Table 6.2), we selected education (again) and caffeine.

What then can we expect about incorporating covariates into the
sleep comparison of AA and CA? Based on the Pearson rs, it is unlikely
that the ANCOVA will gain power. As for equating groups on the
covariates, the low rs will likely also reduce the meaningfulness of this
exercise. We nevertheless proceeded to test the usefulness of ANCOVA.

Ethnicity and Sleep

As we did in chapter 5, we collapsed age into young (20–69 years) and
old (70–89 + years) groups to preserve a reliable cell sample size. We performed a two-factor MANOVA, 2 age groups × 2 ethnic groups, for
seven sleep measures, SOL, NWAK, WASO, TST, SE, SQR, and NAP.
The main effects for age, Wilks' $\Lambda = 0.88, F(7, 583) = 10.94, p < .001$,
and ethnicity, Wilks' $\Lambda = 0.86, F(7, 583) = 13.41, p < .001$, and their interaction, Wilks' $\Lambda = 0.96, F(7, 583) = 3.71, p < .01$, attained significance. Table 6.3 presents means (and SDs) for sleep measures by age and
ethnicity. The parallel covariate analyses, as expected, mirrored the
findings just described. The MANCOVA results were identical to the
MANOVA. The univariate ANCOVA results and the adjusted means
showed only minor variation from the ANOVAs, and therefore the results of the covariate analyses are not reported here.

As would be expected, univariate analyses following the MANOVA
produced significant main effects for age and ethnicity and their interaction. Considering the interaction first, SE and TST produced significant
interactions, and these results are indicated in Table 6.3. In brief, for SE,

TABLE 6.3

Mean and SD Comparing Sleep Measures in Young and Older AA and CA in the Broad Normal Sample

| | Younger Adults (Ages 20–69) | | | | Older Adults (Ages 70–89+) | | | |
| | AA | | CA | | AA | | CA | |
Variable	M	SD	M	SD	M	SD	M	SD
SOL	23.5	15.8	15.5	10.7	24.9	13.8	18.9	14.1
NWAK	1.1	0.9	1.3	0.9	1.5	1.2	1.7	0.9
WASO	20.3	24.5	14.8	15.3	21.3	16.8	24.3	22.6
TST[b,c]	412.8	72.6	424.8	51.9	481.4	75.2	432.8	63.2
Se[a,d]	85.6	8.5	90.3	5.7	86.6	7.3	87.6	6.3
SQR	3.5	0.7	3.6	0.6	3.6	0.6	3.6	0.7
NAP	20.2	22.5	11.6	18.2	34.0	24.1	18.0	21.5

[a]There is a significant difference ($p < .05$) in means comparing AA to CA in the Young group.
[b]There is a significant difference ($p < .05$) in means comparing AA to CA in the Old group.
[c]There is a significant difference ($p < .05$) in means comparing AA in the Young and Old groups.
[d]There is a significant difference ($p < .05$) in means comparing CA in the Young and Old groups.

the Young CA group produced a high SE (90.3%) that distinguished it from same-aged AA and both older groups. A different pattern emerged for TST. Here, Old AA reported the longest TST, about 8 h, among the four cells. Figures 6.1 and 6.2 portray the SE and TST results.

Main effects for age in the broad normal sample are analyzed in chapter 4 and are not repeated here. For the ethnicity factor, in addition to SE and TST contributing to the interaction, univariate main effects were found for SOL and NAP. On the average, AA took longer to fall asleep ($M = 23.7$ min, $SD = 15.5$) than CA ($M = 16.5$, $SD = 11.8$), and AA napped more ($M = 22.7$ min, $SD = 23.3$) than CA ($M = 13.3$, $SD = 19.3$).

Summary. Young CA have better SE than young AA, and old AA have greater TST than old CA. Irrespective of age, CA fall asleep faster (SOL) and nap less than AA. The SE and SOL findings clearly speak to better reported sleep for CA. The TST and NAP findings are more difficult to interpret. We investigated eight explanatory variables, but covariate analyses could not account for differences in AA and CA sleep.

Combining TST and NAP data, CA reported sleeping on the average 7.5 h per 24 h period. Most sleep clinicians would probably consider this

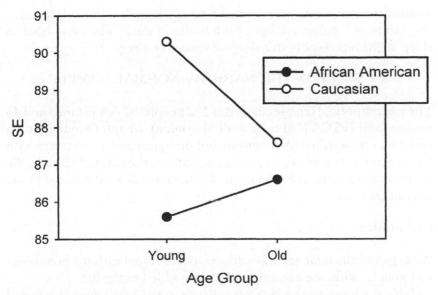

FIG. 6.1.   The age × ethnicity interaction for sleep efficiency percent in the broad normal sample. This interaction was accounted for mainly by higher SE among CA in the young group.

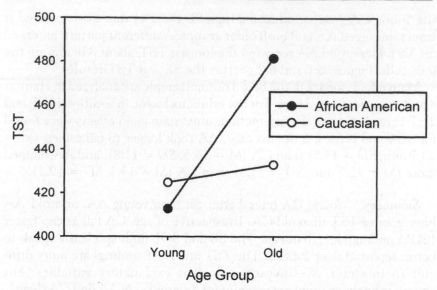

FIG. 6.2.   The age × ethnicity interaction for total sleep time in minutes in the broad normal sample. This interaction was accounted for mainly by the sharp increase in TST in older AA.

a satisfactory amount. AA reported 8.6 h of sleep. It is difficult to judge the merits of a group average of 8.6 hours of sleep. The extra hour of sleep might represent better sleep or excessive sleep.

AA SLEEP IN THE NARROW NORMAL SAMPLE

The narrow normal sample comprises 392 people, 97 AA (51 men and 46 women) and 295 CA (161 men and 134 women). Chapter 4 found a main effect for ethnicity in this subgroup, but no significant interactions with age or gender. Therefore, we proceed to explore the main effect only. We begin with the same consideration of covariates as we did in the broad normal sample.

Covariates

We explored the same set of covariates as was tested with the broad normal sample, with one exception: Age was added to the list.

Table 6.4 presents the Pearson *r*s between the nine covariates tested and SE. In contrast to the broad normal sample, we now find none of the *r*s even reached the .1 level and none were significant.

TABLE 6.4

Pearson Correlation Between Sleep Efficiency Percent and Plausibly Related Demographics in the Narrow Normal Sample

Demographic	n^a	r
Gender[b]	392	–.06
Age	392	–.04
Education	330	.08
BMI	390	–.05
Illness count	392	–.08
Medication count	392	–.05
Caffeine	390	.05
Cigarettes	390	.05
Alcohol	391	.00

[a]Variations in n are due to missing data.
[b]By our coding scheme, the negative correlation reflects better sleep for men.

We next performed t-tests comparing the two ethnic groups on each of these variables excepting for the nominal variable gender. These results are given in Table 6.5. Significant differences were found for six of eight variables. CA had an advantage with significantly higher education and lower BMI. AA had an advantage with significantly lower number of medications used, caffeine and alcohol consumption, and cigarettes smoked. Two of the comparisons registered moderate effect sizes, education and caffeine. Effect size was computed only for significant variables. Although we would have preferred that these two variables be also strongly correlated with sleep, we did enlist education and caffeine as covariates. The comparison of gender distribution by ethnic group proved nonsignificant, $\chi^2(1, N = 392) = 0.12, ns$.

Ethnicity and Sleep

We performed a one-factor MANOVA comparing the two ethnic groups, for seven sleep measures, SOL, NWAK, WASO, TST, SE, SQR,

TABLE 6.5

Comparison of AA and CA on Potential Covariates
in the Narrow Normal Sample

| Variable | AA | | CA | | |
	M	SD	M	SD	d^a
Age	48.5	19.3	51.3	19.0	
Education***	13.4	3.3	15.0	2.5	−0.61
BMI**	27.8	5.8	25.6	4.8	−0.43
Illness count	0.8	1.1	0.8	1.1	
Medication count*	1.3	2.0	1.8	1.9	0.25
Caffeine***	1.3	1.3	2.7	2.6	0.56
Cigarettes**	2.1	5.5	4.7	10.4	0.28
Alcohol*	1.9	3.6	3.0	5.6	0.22

^{a}Positive signs reflect favorably on AA and negative signs reflect favorably on CA. *$p < .05$. **$p < .01$. ***$p < .001$.

and NAP. Ethnicity proved significant, Wilks' $\Lambda = 0.87$, $F(7, 384) = 8.16$, $p < .001$. Table 6.6 presents means (and SDs) for sleep measures by ethnicity. As with the broad normal sample, the covariate analyses produced results virtually identical to the MANOVA, and therefore, the findings of the MANCOVA are not reported.

Significant univariate results were found for SOL, NWAK, SE, and NAP, although only one, NAP, approached a medium effect size. There was no significant difference between AA and CA on three variables, WASO, TST, and SQR. Three of the variables for which there was a significant difference indicated better sleep for CA, SOL, SE, and NAP (assuming more nap time is undesirable). AA reported significantly fewer awakenings during the night than CA, but this was the smallest effect size.

Summary. In the narrow normal sample, CA sleep better than AA, but the magnitude of the difference is not great. On about half the sleep variables, there was either no significant difference or AA slept better by a small margin. Three of the four variables that did show a significant dif-

TABLE 6.6
Mean and SD Comparing Sleep Measures in AA and CA
in the Narrow Normal Sample

| Variable | AA | | CA | | |
	M	SD	M	SD	d^a
SOL***	17.0	8.2	13.4	8.6	−0.42
NWAK**	0.9	0.9	1.3	0.9	0.37
WASO	9.7	9.7	11.3	8.8	
TST	434.4	71.5	432.9	53.9	
SE**	90.0	4.7	91.6	4.0	−0.38
SQR	3.7	0.6	3.7	0.6	
NAP***	19.5	21.3	11.2	15.2	−0.49

^{a}Positive signs reflect favorably on AA and negative signs reflect favorably on CA. **p < .01.
***p < .001.

ference favored the sleep of CA, but only NAP exhibited a meaningful magnitude. Similar to the broad normal sample, we investigated nine explanatory variables, but covariate analyses could not account for differences in AA and CA sleep.

INSOMNIA PREVALENCE BY ETHNICITY

Of the 136 people with insomnia (PWI) identified in chapter 5, 40 were AA (29.4%) and 96 CA (70.6%). This distribution closely matches the relative prevalence of all AA and CA in our sample (see chap. 3). The gender distribution within ethnicity was lopsided, but failed to reach significance, $\chi^2(1, N = 136) = 2.57$, ns. There were 12 AA men (30%) and 28 AA women (70%), and 43 CA men (45%) and 53 CA women (55%). Much of the gender imbalance in insomnia reported in chapter 5 is attributed to AA.

Relating these occurrences of insomnia to the ethnic breakdown in the full sample (762 participants) used in chapter 5, the prevalence of insomnia is 17.9% among AA and 17.8% among CA. Again, these figures do not fairly reflect insomnia prevalence in the general population because we oversampled older adults. Although these rates are probably overstated for the general population, we can nonetheless conclude that the prevalence of insomnia in AA and CA is virtually identical.

Table 6.7 presents the frequency distribution of insomnia by ethnicity across age groups. Although the overall prevalence of insomnia among AA and CA is the same, the distribution of insomnia in AA and CA significantly differed across age groups, $\chi^2(6, N = 136) = 16.64, p < .05$.

The prevalence columns of Table 6.7 divide the observed frequency of PWI by their respective number of participants within ethnic group by decade to determine insomnia prevalence by decade and ethnicity. Among CA, prevalence of insomnia gradually rises over the life span as is customarily observed in epidemiological studies (see chap. 2). However, AA prevalence showed a distinctive pattern across decades. This can be more clearly seen in Fig. 6.3. Peaks in insomnia among AA occur in the middle years, decades 30, 40, and 50, and then again in decades 70 and 80. Except for low levels in decades 20 and 60, insomnia prevalence among AA is flat across the life span.

TABLE 6.7
Prevalence of Insomnia by Ethnicity

	Frequency		Prevalence[a]	
Age	AA	CA	AA	CA
20–29	3	6	2.4% (41)	9.8% (61)
30–39	11	8	23.4% (47)	11.1% (72)
40–49	7	9	20.6% (34)	12.7% (71)
50–59	7	11	21.9% (32)	13.1% (84)
60–69	3	11	11.1% (27)	13.9% (79)
70–79	3	24	18.8% (16)	25.3% (95)
80–89+	6	27	22.2% (26)	35.1% (77)
Total	40	96	(223)	(539)

[a]Prevalence by decade. The insomnia frequency in each decade is affected by the number of AA and CA present in the sample in that decade. Insomnia frequency for AA and CA is referenced to the total number of AA and CA in each decade (given in parentheses) to produce age-based prevalence estimates.

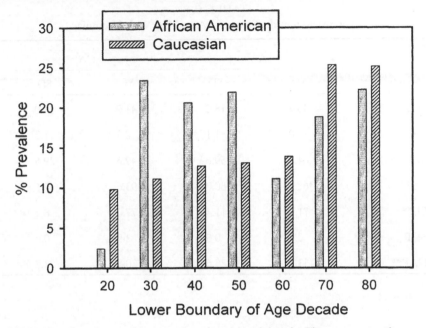

FIG. 6.3. Prevalence of insomnia by ethnicity and decade. There was a significant difference in the distribution of these two groups. CA exhibit the familiar increase in insomnia prevalence across the life span and AA reveal a level pattern except for dips in decades 20 and 60.

INSOMNIA: MAIN EFFECTS OF ETHNICITY

Considering the seven sleep measures, the main effect for ethnicity proved significant, Wilks' Λ = 0.82, $F(7, 128)$ = 3.91, $p < .01$. Univariate follow-up testing revealed that mean AA sleep was worse than CA on all variables except NWAK. Significant differences were found on three variables, TST, SE, and NAP (Table 6.8).

A closer examination of SE illuminates the discrepancy between AA and CA PWI. SE is probably the best single measure that represents the general sleep experience because it reflects several of the other sleep measures, including SOL, WASO, and TST. Figure 6.4 plots SE in these two ethnic groups by decade. The sleep of AA PWI is worse in every decade except decade 20. In four decades, 40, 60, 70, and 80, the difference is about 10 percentage points.

In summary, the data present a consistent view of ethnic differences in insomnia severity. Insomnia is more severe in AA.

TABLE 6.8
Comparison of the Sleep of AA and CA With Insomnia

Variable	AA		CA	
	M	SD	M	SD
SOL	45.7	18.0	41.0	27.0
NWAK	2.0	1.1	2.3	1.2
WASO	64.1	59.6	49.6	29.5
TST*	361.2	80.0	393.6	67.6
SE**	71.7	11.3	77.0	8.2
SQR	2.7	0.5	2.9	0.6
NAP**	33.1	28.6	20.8	22.2

*$p < .05$. **$p < .01$.

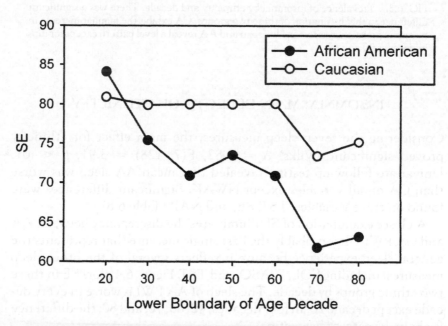

FIG. 6.4.   Sleep efficiency percent by ethnicity and decade among people with insomnia. There was a significant difference in SE between AA and CA.

Covariates

We engaged the same exploration of explanatory variables as we did in the two normal samples. Supplementing the nine variables previously considered, we added two covariates specific to insomnia, years duration of insomnia and number of nights during the 2 weeks of sleep data collection that the participant used sleeping pills.

Table 6.9 presents the Pearson rs for the 11 potential covariates and SE. Three variables were significant, age, education, and illness count, and in all three instances, the r was at or above our original criterion for selecting covariates.

TABLE 6.9
Pearson Correlation Between Sleep Efficiency Percent and Plausibly
Related Demographics in People with Insomnia

Demographic	n^a	r	r^2
Gender[b]	136	−.09	.01
Age	136	−.25**	.06
Education	119	.41***	.16
BMI	136	.02	0
Illness count	136	−.20*	.04
Medication count	136	−.12	.01
Caffeine	136	.10	.01
Cigarettes	136	−.08	.01
Alcohol	135	.08	.01
Duration insomnia	136	−.06	0
Number of sleep medication nights	136	.03	0

[a]Variations in n are due to missing data.
[b]By our coding scheme, the negative correlation reflects better sleep for men. *$p < .05$. **$p < .01$. ***$p < .001$.

Table 6.10 presents *t*-tests comparing AA and CA PWI on 10 of the covariates. Age and education were significant, and both registered medium effect sizes. We did not compute effect size for nonsignificant variables. AA PWI in our sample were younger than CA PWI, but were also less educated. The gender distribution by ethnic group was nonsignificant, $\chi^2(1, N = 136) = 2.57, ns$.

This is the first analysis to identify robust covariates. Age and education met both our criteria for inclusion, and illness count met one. We include all three.

MANCOVA of Main Effects of Ethnicity Among PWI

We immediately encountered a problem due to missing data occurring with the covariates. When the three covariates were added to the MANOVA model, the sample size dropped from 136 (40 AA and 96

TABLE 6.10
Comparison of AA and CA People With Insomnia on Potential Covariates

Variable	AA		CA		
	M	SD	M	SD	d^a
Age***	51.2	18.3	64.4	19.4	0.69
Education**	12.2	2.5	13.9	2.8	−0.63
BMI	28.1	6.0	26.7	6.4	
Illness count	2.0	1.6	2.3	1.7	
Medication count	2.8	2.6	3.7	2.9	
Caffeine	2.2	2.6	2.3	2.9	
Cigarettes	4.8	10.6	3.9	10.0	
Alcohol	1.2	2.5	2.1	5.6	
Duration insomnia	9.3	11.4	9.4	11.5	
Number of sleep medication nights	4.5	6.0	4.9	5.7	

[a]Positive signs reflect favorably on AA and negative signs reflect favorably on CA. **$p < .01$. ***$p < .001$.

CA) to 119 (35 AA and 84 CA). As a result, we are unable to compare the results from the MANCOVA with the original MANOVA because they are analyzing different data sets separated by 17 participants. We considered several remedial strategies to resolve this disparity. In our opinion, the most reasonable solution is to retain the original MANOVA results derived from the largest sample size, but to also redo the MANOVA and MANCOVA on the smaller sample size to fairly contrast the two procedures.

MANOVA and MANCOVA on 119 PWI. The MANOVA comparing AA and CA PWI on the seven sleep measures was significant, Wilks' $\Lambda = 0.85$, $F(7, 111) = 2.79$, $p < .05$. Univariate follow-up testing revealed that mean AA sleep was worse than CA on all variables except NWAK (Table 6.11). We previously found significant differences on three variables, TST, SE, and NAP. We now find these three variables are still significant, as is a fourth, SQR. In sum, the current results substantially replicated the MANOVA on 136 PWI.

The MANCOVA, controlling for age, education, and illness count, comparing AA and CA PWI on the seven sleep measures was also signifi-

TABLE 6.11
Comparison of the Sleep of AA and CA With Insomnia, Sample of 119

| Variable | AA | | CA | |
	M	SD	M	SD
SOL	43.7	16.6	42.2	28.1
NWAK	2.0	0.9	2.2	1.2
WASO	60.1	52.8	49.1	30.7
TST*	363.6	78.0	393.3	70.0
SE*	72.7	11.0	76.8	8.5
SQR*	2.7	0.6	3.0	0.6
NAP*	32.8	28.8	21.5	22.4

*$p < .05$.

cant, Wilks' $\Lambda = 0.86, F(7, 108) = 2.52, p < .05$. At the univariate level, nonsignificant differences between ethnic groups on SOL and NWAK persisted as they have on all ethnic PWI tests. We focus on adjusted means derived from univariate ANCOVAs on the remaining five sleep measures (Table 6.12).

Comparing the adjusted means to the raw means in the sample of 119 (Table 6.11), the ANCOVA expanded the differences between means on three measures, WASO, SE, and NAP, and shrank the difference between means on two measures, TST and SQR. In all cases, the direction of the difference was unchanged. AA faired worse on all five of the adjusted sleep measures, as they have in the two previous analyses.

ANCOVA determined that significant differences occurred on three measures, WASO, SE, and NAP. Compared to the original MANOVA, where three significant differences were also found, there has been a shift. SE and NAP were significant in both analyses. The original MANOVA found TST was significant, and the current analysis found WASO was significant. The MANOVA on the sample of 119 found four significant differences. Adding to SE and NAP in the MANCOVA, it found TST and SQR to be significant. These two results were lost in the MANCOVA, but significance for WASO was added.

TABLE 6.12

Comparison of the Sleep of AA and CA With Insomnia, ANCOVA
Adjusted Means in the Sample of 119

Variable	AA		CA	
	M	SD	M	SD
WASO*	64.1	6.5	47.4	4.0
TST	366.8	13.4	392.0	8.2
SE*	72.2	1.5	77.0	0.9
SQR	2.7	0.1	2.9	0.1
NAP**	35.2	4.5	20.6	2.7

$*p < .05. **p < .01.$

The summary finding from the MANOVA observed that insomnia is more severe in AA than CA. This conclusion is unchanged by the MANCOVA.

INSOMNIA: THE AGE × GENDER × ETHNICITY INTERACTION

Chapter 5 did not test the age × gender × ethnicity interaction on the set of sleep measures because there was an insufficient number of participants to supply all of the cells. The problem of N can be inferred from Table 6.7. When you distribute 40 AA PWI across two levels of gender and seven levels of age, you average fewer than 3 participants per cell.

We wish to explore the interaction of ethnicity with these other factors as best we can. The only feasible way of doing this is to separately explore the age × ethnicity and the gender × ethnicity interactions across fewer than seven levels of age. As we did in chapter 5, we collapsed age into young (20–69 years) and old (70–89+ years) groups. This dichotomy results in 31 young AA PWI and 9 old AA PWI. Although these numbers are not as great as we would prefer, we believe they are sufficient to perform reliable analyses. The numbers for CA PWI are greater and more balanced: 45 young and 51 old.

Age × Ethnicity Interaction

The age × ethnicity MANOVA on the set of sleep measures yielded significant main effects for age, Wilks' $\Lambda = 0.75$, $F(7, 126) = 6.03$, $p < .001$, and ethnicity, Wilks' $\Lambda = 0.76$, $F(7, 126) = 5.97$, $p < .001$, and their interaction, Wilks' $\Lambda = 0.90$, $F(7, 126) = 2.11$, $p < .05$ (Table 6.13). At the univariate level, four variables produced significant main effects for age, NWAK, WASO, SE, and NAP (these results are similar but not identical to the one factor comparison of young and old PWI reported in chap. 5, see Table 5.5); five variables produced significant main effects for ethnicity, WASO, TST, SE, SQR, and NAP (these results are similar but not identical to the one factor comparison of AA and CA PWI reported earlier in this chapter; see Table 6.8); and three variables produced significant age × ethnicity interactions, SOL, WASO, and SQR.

To pursue the analysis of simple effects for the interaction on the three variables just noted, we compared ethnic groups within age levels and we compared age levels within ethnic groups. We will report only significant findings. Cell means and SDs used for these analyses are presented in Table 6.13.

TABLE 6.13

Mean and SD Comparing Sleep Measures in AA and CA With Insomnia in Young and Older Age Groups

| | Younger Adults: Ages 20–69 | | | | Older Adults: Ages 70–89+ | | | |
| | AA | | CA | | AA | | CA | |
Variable	M	SD	M	SD	M	SD	M	SD
SOL*	48.1	18.4	34.7	17.4	37.5	14.4	46.5	32.5
NWAK†	1.8	1.1	2.2	1.3	2.6	0.9	2.4	1.2
WASO†††‡‡‡*	51.2	48.2	40.8	23.4	108.7	75.5	57.3	32.3
TST‡	367.6	72.1	395.7	61.7	339.1	105.1	391.7	72.9
SE†††‡‡	74.4	9.5	80.1	6.4	62.7	13.0	74.4	8.7
SQR‡*	2.8	0.6	2.8	0.6	2.4	0.3	3.0	0.5
NAP†‡‡	30.4	27.5	15.9	16.2	42.2	32.3	25.2	25.8

†Significant main effect for age, p < .05. ‡Significant main effect for age, p < .05. ‡‡Significant main effect for ethnicity, p < .01. ‡‡‡Significant main effect for ethnicity, p < .05.

†Significant main effect for age, p < .05. ††Significant main effect for ethnicity, p < .001. ‡‡‡Significant main effect for ethnicity, p < .05. *Significant interaction effect, p < .05.

For the simple effects of age, old AA scored worse than young AA on WASO and SQR. Old CA scored worse than young CA on SOL and WASO. For the simple effects of ethnicity, among young PWI, AA had greater SOL than CA. Among old PWI, AA scored worse than CA on SQR.

These complex relationships are made clearer by figural presentation (Figs. 6.5, 6.6, and 6.7). Further clarification is needed with regard to Figure 6.5. Although the change in AA SOL appears dramatic, only the AA–CA comparison in the young group reached significance. Neither the decrease in AA SOL across age groups nor the AA–CA comparison in the old group was significant. In summary, older AA sleep worse than young AA on two (WASO and SQR) of three measures. Older CA also sleep worse than young CA on two (SOL and WASO) of three measures. Young AA sleep worse than young CA on one measure, SOL. Old AA also sleep worse than old CA on one measure, SQR.

Gender × Ethnicity Interaction

The number of AA men (12) and women (28) PWI showed greater imbalance than CA men (43) and women (53), although these differences in gender distribution failed to reach significance, $\chi^2(1, N = 136) = 2.65, p = .11$. Women account for 70% of AA PWI but only 55% of CA

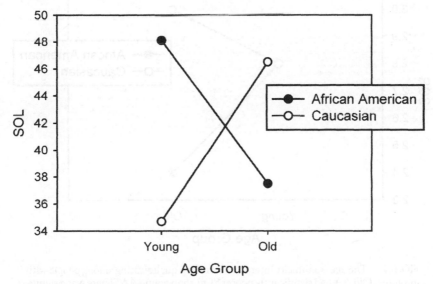

FIG. 6.5.   The age × ethnicity interaction for sleep onset latency in minutes among people with insomnia. There was a significant difference between AA and CA in the young group. Old CA had significantly longer SOL than young CA.

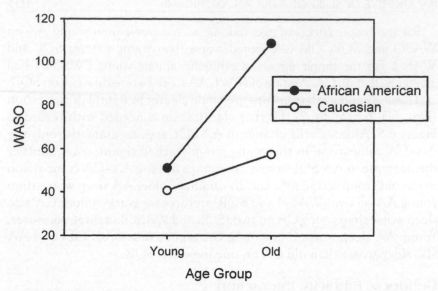

FIG. 6.6. The age × ethnicity interaction for wake time after sleep onset in minutes among people with insomnia. Old AA and CA had significantly longer WASO than young AA and CA.

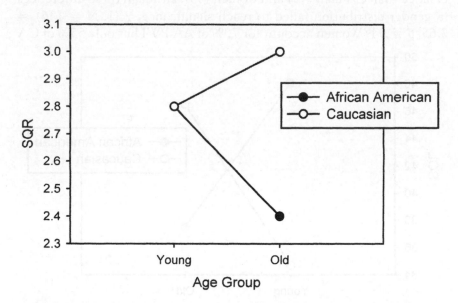

FIG. 6.7. The age × ethnicity interaction for sleep quality rating among people with insomnia. Old AA had significantly poorer SQR than young AA. There was a significant difference between AA and CA in the old group.

PWI. AA women contribute heavily to the significant difference in gen-der prevalence in PWI reported in chapter 5.

We performed a two-factor MANOVA, gender × ethnicity, for the seven sleep measures. Neither the main effect for gender, Wilks' Λ = 0.95, $F(7, 126)$ = 0.99, nor the gender × ethnicity interaction, Wilks' Λ = 0.91, $F(7, 126)$ = 1.83, attained significance. The gender results mir-ror the findings associated with this factor in PWI in chapter 5.

Consistent with the results reported earlier in this chapter, the main effect for ethnicity was significant, Wilks' Λ = 0.82, $F(7, 126)$ = 3.89, $p < .01$.

ETHNICITY AND DAYTIME FUNCTIONING

Broad Normal Sample

We have six daytime functioning measures: Epworth Sleepiness Scale (ESS), Stanford Sleepiness Scale, modified from state to trait (SSS), Fa-tigue Severity Scale (FSS), Insomnia Impact Scale (IIS), Beck Depres-sion Inventory (BDI), and State Trait Anxiety Inventory, trait form (STAI). The MANOVA comparing AA and CA on this set of measures proved significant, Wilks' Λ = 0.96, $F(6, 586)$ = 4.57, $p < .001$.

AA exhibited poorer functioning on every measure, and the differ-ence was significant on all but one, FSS (Table 6.14). We then consid-ered criteria for clinical meaningfulness of these scores based on cutoffs we have previously justified (Lichstein, Durrence, Taylor, Bush, & Riedel, 2003). It is important to note that, with the possible exception of ESS, none of the means were in the pathological range. Clear cutoffs for excessive daytime sleepiness on the ESS do not exist.

Narrow Normal Sample

The MANOVA comparing AA and CA on the set of daytime function-ing measures (ESS, SSS, FSS, IIS, BDI, and STAI) proved significant, Wilks' Λ = 0.97, $F(6, 385)$ = 2.33, $p < .05$. Again, AA exhibited poorer functioning on every measure, but in contrast to the broad normal sam-ple, the difference was significant on only two, ESS and BDI (Table 6.15). Here too, none of the means were in the pathological range (Lichstein et al., 2003), and in general, the scores dropped more deeply into the normal range compared to the broad normal sample.

TABLE 6.14

Mean and SD Comparing Daytime Functioning Measures in AA and CA
in the Broad Normal Sample

Variable	AA		CA	
	M	SD	M	SD
ESS***	9.4	4.5	8.0	3.8
SSS*	3.0	1.7	2.6	1.4
FSS	3.5	1.4	3.3	1.2
IIS**	102.0	23.7	95.9	22.3
BDI***	8.7	7.6	6.4	5.7
STAI**	36.3	10.3	33.6	9.3

*$p < .05$. **$p < .01$. ***$p < .001$.

TABLE 6.15

Mean and SD Comparing Daytime Functioning Measures in AA and CA
in the Narrow Normal Sample

Variable	AA		CA	
	M	SD	M	SD
ESS*	8.9	4.2	7.8	3.8
SSS	2.8	1.7	2.5	1.3
FSS	3.2	1.4	3.2	1.2
IIS	95.3	23.1	94.2	21.4
BDI**	7.0	6.6	5.2	4.8
STAI	34.3	10.5	32.7	8.8

*$p < .05$. **$p < .01$.

People With Insomnia

The MANOVA comparing AA and CA PWI proved significant, Wilks' $\Lambda = 0.87$, $F(6, 129) = 3.19$, $p < .01$. Consistent with the findings in the normal sleeping samples, AA exhibited greater impairment on all measures but one, FSS (Table 6.16). As with the narrow normal sample, significant differences occurred with only two measures, IIS and STAI, although not the same two as in the narrow normal sample.

Not surprisingly, daytime functioning scores in the PWI sample did become clinically meaningful (Lichstein et al., 2003). The ESS scores in both groups and the IIS score in the AA group approached pathological levels. The BDI and STAI means for both AA and CA were in the clinically significant range.

TABLE 6.16
**Mean and SD Comparing Daytime Functioning Measures
in AA and CA People With Insomnia**

| Variable | AA | | CA | |
	M	SD	M	SD
ESS	10.2	4.6	9.6	4.5
SSS	3.9	1.6	3.7	1.5
FSS	4.3	1.4	4.4	1.3
IIS*	121.5	28.9	111.8	22.8
BDI	15.5	10.8	13.2	8.1
STAI***	48.9	9.4	41.3	11.5

*$p < .05$. ***$p < .001$.

7

Summary of Main Findings

After collecting so much information and conducting so many analyses, what has this data set taught us about people's self-perceptions of their sleep? Chapters 4, 5, and 6 answer this question and provide the framework for this chapter. Thus, the main sections of this chapter explore normal sleep, insomnia, and the sleep of African Americans (AA). In each section, we attempt to organize the primary findings of this project by addressing the following points:

- Main findings that confirm existing beliefs.
- Main findings that contradict existing beliefs.
- Novel findings from this survey.

For reasons described later, we depart from this structure in the section on sleep of AA.

NORMAL SLEEP

Much of the inspiration for this epidemiological survey derived from our previous work that was limited by its dependence on the restricted availability of self-reported sleep norms for normal sleepers (Lichstein, 1997). Our inability to locate adequate norms convinced us of the need to conduct the present survey. "There is a large amount of existing polysomnography (PSG) data for normal sleepers and people with insomnia, and there is a large amount of existing self-reported sleep data for people with insomnia. But there is a small amount of existing self-reported sleep data for normal sleepers" (Lichstein, 1997, p. 1136). What little data exist come from either nonrandom, convenience samples, surveys targeting restricted segments of the commu-

202

nity, or surveys collecting limited amounts of information. The scant availability of this type of data forced our epidemiology review (chap. 2) to focus only on insomnia. Nearly all the data collected in the present normal sleeping samples are novel data.

We were befuddled at the very outset of data analysis when our group couldn't agree on who met the definition of normal sleep. The problem is that there are many such definitions, and legitimate arguments can be advanced in behalf of all of them. First, from the bell-curve perspective, normalcy includes the tails of the distribution, suggesting that the entire sample represented the range of normalcy. Second, we considered that normal sleep refers to the absence of pathological sleep, and we excluded from our sample those who reported sleep disorders such as apnea and periodic limb movements and those who satisfied our definition of insomnia. We called this the broad normal sample. Third, we thought it would be useful to define normal sleep more narrowly, equating the terms normal and desirable. We eliminated from the broad normal sample individuals who complained of insomnia but did not satisfy our quantitative criteria and individuals who did satisfy our quantitative criteria for insomnia but did not perceive themselves as having insomnia, sometimes referred to as noncomplaining poor sleepers in the insomnia literature. This group, termed the narrow normal sample, would present a portrait of perfectly healthy sleep, representing the goal limits for those dissatisfied with their sleep. We settled on the second and third definitions and analyzed these two groups separately. However, we did present tables of sleep norms for all three groups.

Main Findings That Confirm Existing Beliefs

As already stated, little is known about self-reported sleep in normal sleepers. Findings summarized in this section as confirming existing beliefs are compared to the small amount of existing data, extrapolation from PSG, or widely held clinical impressions.

Broad Normal Sample. It is a truism that older adults sleep worse than younger adults, but this proved out only in a minority of our sleep measures. Number of awakenings during the night (NWAK), wake time after sleep onset (WASO), and time spent napping (NAP) all got worse in the later years. This conclusion assumes increased NAP reflects negatively on sleep, which may not be true in a retired population. Excluding NAP for the moment, older adults' self-reported sleep was worse than younger adults' on two of six measures.

What influences would account for fragmented sleep (NWAK and WASO) in older adults that would not also degrade other aspects of sleep? Some combination of three factors could plausibly explain this pattern. First, sleep apnea and periodic limb movements rise dramatically in older adults (Ancoli-Israel et al., 1991a, 1991b) and would contribute to difficulty sustaining sleep. Second, the distribution of sleep stages in older adults differs from younger people. Decreased deep sleep, stages 3 and 4, and increased light sleep, stage 2 (Morgan, 2000), would increase vulnerability to awakenings during the night. Third, nocturia is more salient in older people (Bliwise, 2000) and could contribute to sleep interruptions.

Narrow Normal Sample. In this sample, we found age effects in the same five sleep variables occurring in the broad normal sample, but three of the variables, NWAK, WASO, and NAP, also contributed to a significant age × gender interaction. Despite the interaction, the results for these three variables mapped closely onto the results for the broad normal sample. They all showed deterioration with advancing age, and there were no consistent differences between men and women of meaningful magnitude.

The remaining variables either showed sleep improvement or no change over the life span. We comment further on these data later.

Main Findings That Contradict Existing Beliefs

Broad Normal Sample. As stated earlier, older adults reported worse sleep on two or three (depending on whether NAP is counted) sleep measures. There was no significant change across the life span on two measures, sleep onset latency (SOL) and sleep efficiency percent (SE), and sleep improved with advancing age on two measures, total sleep time (TST) and sleep quality rating (SQR).

These data are surprising in three respects. First, the oldest group reported the greatest TST. Others, based mainly on PSG data, have reported a decline in TST with advancing age (Bixler & Vela-Bueno, 1987; Feinberg & Carlson, 1968; Kupfer & Reynolds, 1983). Interestingly, in a nonrandom sleep survey, Webb (1965) found an increase in self-reported TST among older adults. A self-report sleep survey of a Dutch town also reported an increase in TST in decade 80 (Middelkoop, Smilde-van den Doel, Neven, Kamphuisen, & Springer, 1996). Second, decade 80 averaged 7.6 h of sleep per night. This was the only decade mean to exceed the customary assumption that normal adults sleep at least 7.5 h per night (Bixler & Vela-Bueno, 1987; Ferrara & De Gennaro, 2001). Third, older adults are pleased with their sleep, as indicated by SQR. Despite increased NWAK and WASO, their view of their sleep experience is on the average more positive than younger adults.

We explored an alternative explanation for why subjective TST would peak in later years. Perhaps older adults' time estimation ability is skewed toward elongation. We reviewed basic research in the developmental literature on time estimation and found no evidence to support the conclusion that greater TST in older adults is a function of time estimation bias. Our SOL data, which were stable across the life span, also refute this explanation. If a time estimation bias were distorting TST, we would assume it would also corrupt SOL.

Our data refute the summary perspective that sleep, or at least the subjective perception of sleep, degenerates in later years. The optimistic tone of our data is consistent with mounting evidence that poor sleep in old age is largely a product of increased prevalence of illness (Lamberg, 2003). The sleep of physically healthy older adults is similar to that of younger adults (Ohayon, 2002). It is possible that our older adult sample was not fairly representative of this segment of the population, in that our sample may have tended to be healthier. This could have been one possible source of bias in our participants. It may be that sickly older adults were less able to tolerate the participant burden of our survey (see discussion in chap. 3) and were less likely to participate.

We found a main effect for gender differences, but these effects were not great. Small-magnitude, statistically significant differences occurred for NWAK, WASO, and SE, and in all three cases, women slept worse than men. There was no significant difference on the majority of measures. These findings conflict with other data reporting that women sleep more than men (Ferrara & De Gennaro, 2001), and there is greater subjective sleep satisfaction among healthy older men compared to older women (Campbell, Gillin, Kripke, Erikson, & Clopton, 1989). Consistent with our findings, one group found little difference in sleep perception between men and women (Voderholzer, Al-Shajlawi, Weske, Feige, & Riemann, 2003). Little else is previously known about the normal self-reported sleep of men and women.

Narrow Normal Sample.   The age findings here are similar to those in the broad normal sample. We have more to say about this in the section that follows on novel findings.

Gender effects are also similar to those in the broad normal sample. The few significant differences reflected better sleep in men, but on the whole, the magnitude of the differences was minor, and the fairest conclusion is that men and women exhibit similar perceptions of their sleep.

Novel Findings From This Survey

Broad Normal Sample. The most important contribution of this survey is to provide self-reported sleep norms for normal sleepers broken down by age, gender, and ethnicity. This information is found in the large appendix to chapter 4. Such normative data have not previously existed. We expect that the utility of these data over the years will find applications difficult to anticipate presently. It is only after such data exist that creative minds will find a use for them. One application that readily comes to mind is using self-reported sleep norms as a standard against which the severity of self-reported insomnia complaints can be judged. Perhaps a metric could be developed (as in Lichstein, 1997) to gauge the summary difference between the two, such that insomnia severity would be proportional to the disparity.

The highest TST (mean = 461.8 min) and the highest NAP (mean = 24.2 min) occurred in decade 80. The total mean sleep time per 24 h period of 486 min, 8.1 h, is second only to the same decade in the narrow normal sample. With SE providing quality control, we cannot endorse the explanation that older adults are devoted to excessive time in bed to acquire greater sleep time. In the context of narrow variation in SE across the seven decades (no significant change), high sleep time appears to reflect greater sleep need in the "old-old" group.

Narrow Normal Sample. What is normal subjective SE? This has not previously been established. Researchers have sometimes used SE as an insomnia criterion, setting it at <85% (Hauri, 1997) or <80% (Bliwise, Friedman, Nekich, & Yesavage, 1995) to qualify. Others (cited in Espie, 1991) have gone as high as <88%. It follows that normal SE is presumed to be higher than these levels. In the broad normal sample, SE did not exceed 90% in any decade. In the narrow normal sample, SE exceeded 90% in every decade, but just barely. Assuming the mean SE closely approximates the median, about half the individuals in the narrow normal sample, that is, the pristine sleepers, reported SE below 90%. It would appear to be unreasonable to conclude that normal SE is 90%. As can be seen in Table 4.8, the SE standard deviation (SD) is greater than 4 in most decades. It would seem reasonable to set the normal SE at least 1 SD below the mean, particularly in the narrow normal sample. We then begin to overlap with insomnia criteria. Perhaps it would be prudent to consider the lower limit of normal SE at 85%. This provides a thin border between normal and abnormal SE and excludes a sizable minority of the narrow normal sample. However, by convention, it would be premature to set normal SE below this point, although later replication of our findings might subsequently justify a lower SE cutoff.

As in the broad normal sample, SOL and SE did not significantly change across the life span. Also, mirroring the broad normal sample, the greatest TST and the peak SQR occurred in the later years. Young adults rated quality of sleep the lowest. Aside from the knowledge that most epidemiological surveys (see chap. 2) agree that insomnia prevalence increases with age, little is known about the experience of normal sleepers. Apparently we can not presume incremental poor sleep in normal sleepers paralleling increased insomnia in older adults. Those who avoid insomnia appear to be preserving important aspects of their sleep from their younger years and, not infrequently, enjoying improved subjective sleep.

Normal Sleep and Daytime Functioning

We jointly discuss the broad and narrow normal samples, because their results were consistent. Similarly, analyses exploring differences by age and gender did not disclose important variation. Further, there is little known about the association between normal sleep and daytime functioning. Therefore, we dispense with the subheading format used in the rest of this chapter because all of this information is novel.

The summary results presented in Table 4.22 serve as the focus of this discussion. Each of our six measures of daytime functioning—Epworth Sleepiness Scale (ESS), Stanford Sleepiness Scale (SSS), Fatigue Severity Scale (FSS), Insomnia Impact Scale (IIS), Beck Depression Inventory (BDI), and State Trait Anxiety Inventory (STAI)—were regressed on the set of seven sleep variables. When collectively referring to the daytime functioning measures, we sometimes use the term *quality of life* to reflect their summary impact.

Perhaps the most distinctive result of these many analyses is that most sleep measures among normal sleepers are insulated from daytime functioning. SOL, NWAK, WASO, and SE showed little relation to the set of daytime functioning indices, which span a broad range of performance

and experience. Knowledge of one's self-reported sleep on these variables did not inform quality of life.

SQR exhibited the strongest relationship to daytime functioning, and
NAP was not far behind. TST registered about half the number of significant associations as NAP, but is considered meaningful because TST
findings were still three to four times more frequent than the four
low-frequency sleep measures cited earlier.

Recalling how our data were collected, participants were instructed
to complete the set of daytime functioning measures at a single sitting
immediately following 2 weeks of sleep diaries. Participants' average ratings of their sleep quality during those 2 weeks were inversely correlated
with quality of life, meaning that better SQR was associated with lower
impairment on the daytime functioning measures. It is interesting to
note that of our seven sleep variables, participants' summary judgment
of their sleep experience was the one most strongly associated with quality of life. Three equally plausible hypotheses may account for the
SQR–daytime functioning relationship. First, poor sleep at night may
have soured next day functioning. Second, the residue of negative daytime experiences may have invaded the following night's sleep. Third,
the relationship between SQR and quality of life may have been
correlational, not causal. Another factor, such as illness or a spell of
hyperarousability (Bonnet & Arand, 1997), or a collection of factors
may have disrupted both sleep and quality of life. The design of this survey precludes favoring any one of these hypotheses.

NAP was also inversely correlated with daytime functioning. More
NAP was consistently associated with poorer quality of life. Here again
we can offer a stream of plausible hypotheses unaccompanied by the ability to determine their relative merits. NAP may be an escape mechanism
from unpleasant days. Choosing to NAP may disrupt the day's flow, interfere with partaking in valued activities, frustrate achievement goals,
or leave the individual with a groggy, negativistic disposition. Illness or
poor sleep the previous night may weaken the individual and instigate
both NAP and degraded quality of life. To obtain greater clarity into the
relationship between both SQR and NAP with quality of life, daily quality of life measures would be required to correspond with the daily sleep
measures. Unfortunately, such data are not available in this study.

Increased TST was associated with diminished quality of life. This
was unexpected but the consistency of this finding bolsters its credibility.
Ordinarily, greater sleep time is welcome, would leave individuals satisfied with their sleep and refreshed, and would do little to impair daytime

functioning. It is possible that some of the same hypotheses proffered to explain the association of increased NAP with diminished quality of life are salient to the TST mechanism as well. Increased TST may be a response to negative events and reflect an individual's desire to prematurely terminate a difficult day. Increased TST may intrude on both daytime (when sleeping late) and nighttime (when going to bed early) activities, curtailing positive experiences and elevating frustration. Fatigue arising from varied sources may facilitate greater TST and also interfere with daytime functioning.

The daytime measures can be rank ordered according to how often we found a significant relationship between a sleep measure and each of them. Starting with the measure most often associated with sleep, the descending sequence is IIS, BDI, FSS, ESS, SSS, and STAI. The IIS samples the broadest range of symptoms and, unlike the BDI, FSS, and STAI, was specifically designed to identify sleep-related problems. Therefore, its sensitivity to sleep variation is not unexpected. Depression (BDI) and fatigue (FSS) have long been associated with poor sleep (Riedel & Lichstein, 2000), so their high ranking is also not unexpected. However, anxiety (STAI) has been shown to have a strong association with poor sleep (Ohayon, 2002), and its last place was not anticipated.

INSOMNIA

Not only did we encounter a problem defining normal sleep, we also felt uncomfortable relying on the *qualitative* diagnostic criteria for insomnia presented in the *Diagnostic and Statistical Manual of Mental Disorders*, 4th edition (*DSM–IV*, American Psychiatric Association, 1994) or the *International Classification of Sleep Disorders: Diagnostic and Coding Manual* (ICSD, American Sleep Disorders Association, 1990). Before we could proceed with the analysis of people with insomnia (PWI), we conducted a study (Lichstein, Durrence, Taylor, Bush, & Riedel, 2003) to derive empirically based, quantitative criteria for identifying the PWI sample. In contrast to most other epidemiological studies of insomnia, having quantitative criteria provided the advantages of being able to specify exactly which people we are studying and to identify insomnia subtypes.

Main Findings That Confirm Existing Beliefs

We found that insomnia is more common in women and more common in older adults. These conclusions echo most epidemiological studies (see chap. 2).

We also found that the severity of insomnia (as measured by NWAK, WASO, and SE) worsens with age, and this also agrees with the thrust of the epidemiological literature (see chap. 2). For PWI, advancing age is ominous. Insomnia is more frequent and more severe in older adults. This is in contrast to our findings for people not having insomnia (PNI), for whom, in the main, advancing age does not bring poorer self-reported sleep.

However, the worsening of insomnia among older adults does not extend to general mood or performance. Our six measures of daytime functioning produced no evidence that this dimension showed greater impairment in older adults.

Comparing poor and good sleepers, PWI were found to have less education, a reliable proxy variable for socioeconomic status (Winkleby, Jatulis, Frank, & Fortmann, 1992). Further, PWI had higher levels of both medical and emotional disorders. All of these findings are consistent with the extant literature (Ohayon, 2002).

We also compared the sleep of PWI and PNI, and the two groups were significantly different on every sleep variable. This outcome was in part determined by using quantitative criteria, rather than global subjective definitions, to assign participants to insomnia or noninsomnia categories. However, it should be acknowledged that PSG sleep evaluations in older adults do not always find significant differences between PWI and PNI (Bastien, LeBlanc, Carrier, & Morin, 2003).

Main Findings That Contradict Existing Beliefs

Chapter 2 did find gender effects for insomnia. Although not completely consistent across studies, women PWI often reported more severe insomnia than men PWI, particularly with respect to SOL and WASO. The present data found no gender effects in the sleep of PWI. Based on the current data, we would conclude that insomnia is more frequent but not more severe in women.

Although there is not a single study that included a broad age distribution of PWI with precision in their definition of insomnia that found onset insomnia mainly occurs in younger adults and maintenance insomnia mainly occurs in older adults, there is a common perception that onset and maintenance insomnia occur unevenly across the life span reflecting this distribution (e.g., Morgan, 2000; Morin, 1993). We (chap. 5) carefully analyzed the prevalence of insomnia types by age and found a small amount of data supporting the view that onset insomnia and maintenance insomnia are primarily associated with young and older adults, respectively. More importantly, the preponderance of our data show that both onset and maintenance insomnia, singly or combined, occur throughout the life span. From a clinical perspective, health providers should be prepared for both onset and maintenance insomnia regardless of the age of their patient.

PWI napped more than PNI in the present sample. Prior research has usually found that PWI and PNI do not significantly differ in napping (Haynes, Adams, West, Kamens, & Safranek, 1982; Lichstein, Durrence, Riedel, & Bayen, 2001; Morin & Gramling, 1989).

Novel Findings From This Survey

We calculated the overall prevalence of insomnia, weighted by gender and age, to be 15.9%. Based on the U.S. census, there are 31.4 million PWI in this country. We consider this prevalence estimate a novel finding because there has never been an insomnia prevalence estimate from an epidemiological study that could rival the methodological rigor of the combination of features of the current study: random-digit dialing sampling, 2 weeks of sleep diaries, quantitative insomnia criteria including daytime impairment, and sampling across a broad age range and across ethnicity. Given the great diversity of survey methods and insomnia prevalence findings in the epidemiology of insomnia literature, there are no comparable estimates.

It is well established that the insomnia prevalence estimate decreases with increasing methodological rigor (Ohayon, 2002). Based on this notion, we were expecting a lower prevalence than we found because we used stringent criteria to diagnose insomnia. Although our survey methods did nothing to attract PWI more so than PNI, it is possible there is a self-selection bias in our data. Perhaps PWI are motivated by greater curiosity about sleep and were more likely to participate. Were there a self-selection bias in our data, we could not say if it was greater or less than that in other epidemiological studies. We have no basis on which to confirm or challenge the self-selection hypothesis. To our knowledge, 15.9% is the best defended prevalence estimate for insomnia.

All of our data on insomnia types are novel. Without the aid of quantitative criteria, previous epidemiological studies were unable to define types with precision. Our four types (defined in chap. 5) are onset, maintenance, mixed, and combined. Maintenance was the most common, but at 31.6%, did not dominate the distribution of types. Mixed was the least common, occurring at about half the rate of maintenance,

16.9%. We should not overlook the finding that there was no statistically significant difference in the prevalence of the four types. Because mixed and combined types include both onset and maintenance, we found that 68% of our sample of PWI had an onset component; they either exclusively experienced onset insomnia or exhibited a mix of onset and maintenance insomnia. Similarly, 77% of our sample experienced maintenance insomnia, either exclusively or co-occurring with onset problems.

Insomnia severity varied by type, but the pattern was not consistent across sleep measures. Typically, maintenance and combined insomnia were more severe than onset and mixed insomnia. However, the four insomnia types did not significantly differ in daytime dysfunction.

Insomnia and Daytime Functioning

The same multiple-regression analyses relating sleep and daytime functioning among PNI were performed with PWI. These results can be efficiently summarized. The relationship between sleep and daytime functioning in PWI is much like that in PNI, weak and inconsistent.

The relationship between sleep and daytime functioning remains clouded. The present data generally found small correlations between night and day experience among both PNI and PWI. It is plausible that the weak association in the normal samples is a function of limited variability in sleep. A restricted range of sleep experience would likely dampen correlations. But there was broader variability in the sleep of PWI. This can be discerned in two tables collapsing across factors, 4.6 and 5.4. PWI have greater variability in every sleep measure, excepting SQR. This greater variability in PWI did not produce stronger sleep–daytime correlations. Based on the present data set, we conclude that sleep and daytime functioning are substantially independent.

Clinical trials could provide a valuable means of clarifying the relationship between daytime and nighttime experience. Observation of the effects of altering daytime functioning on sleep as well as the effects of changing sleep on daytime functioning could illuminate these complex relationships. Half of this data source is missing. We are unaware of any study that tested sleep effects of intervening on daytime functioning. There are many clinical trials that treated insomnia and measured daytime functioning, but these results are inconsistent. Some studies have reported improved daytime functioning following insomnia improvement (Backhaus, Hohagen, Voderholzer, & Riemann,

2001; Morin, Kowatch, Barry, & Walton, 1993; Shealy, Lowe, & Ritzler, 1980) and some have not observed improved daytime functioning after successful insomnia treatment (Lichstein, Riedel, Wilson, Lester, & Aguillard, 2001; Means, Lichstein, Epperson, & Johnson, 2000; Morin & Azrin, 1988).

Presumably, for some individuals at some period in their life, sleep change instigates corresponding alterations in quality of life, and similarly, fluctuations in daytime functioning induce isomorphic sleep change. However, group analyses may conceal individual differences in this area. For the present, the following summary conclusions fairly capture the current state of knowledge for both PNI and PWI.

- The association between sleep and daytime functioning is usually weak.
- When corresponding change does occur, the direction of the causal path from day influencing night or from night influencing day is unclear.
- The factors responsible for causal links between night and day experience are not known and are not replicable.

THE SLEEP OF AFRICAN AMERICANS

This segment of the U.S. population has been under studied by sleep researchers. Nearly everything we learned about the sleep of AA in the present study is novel. When comparable data do exist, the number of extant studies is small. Therefore, we dispensed with the tripartite structure of this chapter for this topic.

Broad Normal Sample

We found an age × ethnicity interaction for SE and TST and main effects for SOL and NAP. Caucasians (CA) reported better sleep in SE, in the young group, and shorter SOL for all ages. CA also reported less NAP than AA, which may be reflective of better nighttime sleep for CA.

The TST findings are a bit harder to interpret. In the older group, AA slept longer than CA. A study of college students agreed with our finding that there was no significant AA–CA difference in TST among young adults (Hicks, Lucero-Gorman, Bautista, & Hicks, 1999). Others in survey (Qureshi, Giles, Croft, & Bliwise, 1997; Schoenborn, 1986) and PSG (Profant, Ancoli-Israel, & Dimsdale, 2002) studies have observed longer TST in AA compared to CA in a broad age range. In contrast, a large epidemiological study of older women found AA women slept about half an hour less than CA women (Kripke et al., 2001).

In our data, CA TST was not inadequate. We cannot determine if the additional TST in older AA represents a health increment or is reflective of increased morbidity (Bliwise, King, & Harris, 1994; Habte-Gabr et al., 1991; Qureshi et al., 1997).

We repeated the tests just described with analysis of covariance (ANCOVA). We modeled six covariables relating to demographics, health, and sleep hygiene, and were unable to explain the described differences.

Narrow Normal Sample

Small-magnitude differences were found on four sleep variables, and three of these (SOL, SE, and NAP) reflected better sleep in CA compared to AA. AA reported fewer NWAK than CA. The TST difference in the broad normal sample did not hold up in the narrow normal sample. A PSG study of small groups of healthy AA and CA with good sleep (Rao, Poland, Lutchmansingh, Ott, McCracken, & Keh-Ming, 1999) also found little to distinguish these groups. They observed no significant difference in any sleep pattern variable: SOL, WASO, TST, or SE. However, differences were found for AA males on sleep architecture variables. This subgroup had more light sleep (stages 1 and 2) and less deep sleep (stage 4) than AA females or CA.

We repeated these tests with ANCOVA. We modeled two co-variables, education level and caffeine consumption, and were unable to explain the described differences.

To summarize the findings for our two normal samples, the differences in sleep between AA and CA are minor. CA perceive their sleep as better than AA on a subset of the sleep variables, but by a small magnitude.

Insomnia

Insomnia prevalence in AA and CA is virtually identical in our sample. This finding is in mild disagreement with that of Karacan, Thornby, Anch, Holzer, Warheit, Schwab, and Williams (1976), who reported a slightly higher rate of insomnia among AA. However, the distribution of insomnia prevalence by age among AA does not follow the gradual ascendancy pattern across the life span commonly observed (chap. 2). AA show a bimodal pattern, with the main peaks occurring in the middle years and peaks occurring again in the late years. Consistent with these findings, two studies (Blazer, Hays, & Foley, 1995; Jean-Louis et al.,

2001) found that AA older adults had fewer sleep complaints than CA older adults. In contrast, Kripke et al. (2001) found little difference in insomnia complaints among older adult AA and CA women.

Adding to the inconsistency of findings in this area, analyses of 3-year follow-up data from the Blazer et al. (1995) survey (Foley, Monjan, Izmirlian, Hays, & Blazer, 1999) amended their previous conclusion. AA women in this older adult sample had a significantly higher incidence of insomnia than either AA men or CA men and women. We also found the highest rate of insomnia in AA women across all ages, but in our sample this did not reach significance.

Significant differences in sleep between AA and CA PWI were found on TST, SE, and NAP, indicating worse sleep for AA, and in contrast to differences occurring in the normal samples, the magnitude of the differences on these three variables was nontrivial. This comparison was subjected to ANCOVA controlling for three covariables, age, education, and illness. With minor variation, this analysis replicated the first.

Exploration of the age × ethnicity sleep interaction among PWI can be summarized briefly. Insomnia severity increases with advancing age on a subset of sleep characteristics. Old AA sleep worse than young AA on WASO and SQR, and old AA sleep worse than old CA on SQR. Not one sleep measure showed significantly better sleep for young AA compared to old AA, or better sleep for AA compared to CA within age groups.

Ethnicity and Daytime Functioning

In both the broad and narrow normal samples, AA reported significantly greater daytime impairment than CA. Two qualifications modify this finding. The difference between AA and CA diminished from the broad normal sample to the narrow normal sample. With minor exception, mean AA scores on our six measures of daytime functioning were not in the pathological range. Among PWI as well, AA showed greater daytime impairment than CA on two measures, IIS and STAI. In sum, these findings are consistent with the thrust of data from the epidemiology of health (Durrence & Lichstein, 2003). AA have poorer health than CA.

CONCLUDING OBSERVATIONS

Perhaps it is fitting to return to the title in closing this book. We can encapsulate the role of age, gender, and ethnicity in self-reported sleep. All three are important sleep factors some of the time.

Among normal sleepers, age is an important factor, but gender and ethnicity are not. Perhaps the experience of advancing age is best captured by the descriptor disorderly: Older adults sleep longer but their sleep is more fragmented. Comparing the sleep of older adults to middle-aged adults, some aspects of sleep are unchanged, some get worse, and some get better. There is greater coherence among the several parts of sleep during the middle-age period. At a minimum, our data do not support the blanket assertion that older adults are condemned to poor sleep.

Age, gender, and ethnicity are all important contributors to understanding insomnia. Insomnia is more frequent in women than men, but not more severe. Insomnia is more frequent in older adults than younger adults, and is more severe in the older group. Insomnia is not more prevalent in AA than CA, but the age distribution in the two groups is dissimilar. Insomnia is more severe in AA than CA.

Using our conservative quantitative criteria and applying a weighted average, we determined the insomnia population prevalence to be 15.9%. This was higher than we anticipated, but perhaps we had been mislead by the existing body of literature on the epidemiology of sleep because of the disarray occurring in the absence of standardized insomnia diagnostic criteria. We also studied type of insomnia: onset, maintenance, mixed, and combined. We did find spikes and droughts of particular types occurring in some age segments, but for the most part, all types are substantially represented in all age groups.

EPILOGUE: THE IRONY OF SLEEP

How can such a common experience be so avoidant of scientific scrutiny? The problem is measurement. A measure of sleep that possesses all the critical elements of unobtrusiveness, objectivity, validity, and reliability has yet to be invented. Each of the available measures can rightfully claim some of these characteristics, but none all. Each measure permits inspection of a dimension of sleep, but none illuminates the complete picture in full blossom. Our present effort focused on subjective experience. It provided another peek into the mystery of sleep, but the phenomenon remains well protected by its indefatigable obscurity.

Appendix A

Alphabetical Listing of Abbreviations and Acronyms

AA	African American(s)
ANCOVA	Analysis of covariance
ANOVA	Analysis of variance
BDI	Beck Depression Inventory
BMI	Body mass index
CA	Caucasian(s)
DSM–IV	Diagnostic and Statistical Manual of Mental Disorders, 4th edition
ESS	Epworth Sleepiness Scale
FSS	Fatigue Severity Scale
ICD-10	International Statistical Classification of Diseases and Related Health Problems, 10th revision
ICSD	International Classification of Sleep Disorders: Diagnostic and Coding Manual
IIS	Insomnia Impact Scale
MANCOVA	Multivariate analysis of covariance
MANOVA	Multivariate analysis of variance
NAP	Time spent napping (minutes)
NWAK	Number of awakenings during the night
PNI	Person or people not having insomnia
PSG	Polysomnography
PWI	Person or people with insomnia
SE	Sleep efficiency percent (TST/TIB × 100)
SOL	Sleep onset latency (minutes)
SQR	Sleep quality rating (1 = very poor, 2 = poor, 3 = fair, 4 = good, and 5 = excellent)
SR	self-report
SSS	Stanford Sleepiness Scale
STAI	State-Trait Anxiety Inventory
TIB	Time in bed
TST	Total sleep time (minutes)
WASO	Wake time after sleep onset (minutes)

References

American Psychiatric Association. (1994). *Diagnostic and statistical manual of mental disorders* (4th ed.). Washington, DC: Author.

American Sleep Disorders Association. (1990). *International classification of sleep disorders: Diagnostic and coding manual*. Rochester, MN: Author.

Ancoli-Israel, S., & Roth, T. (1999). Characteristics of insomnia in the United States: Results of the 1991 National Sleep Foundation Survey. I. *Sleep, 22* (Suppl. 2), S347–S353.

Ancoli-Israel, S., Kripke, D. F., Klauber, M. R., Mason, W. J., Fell, R., & Kaplan, O. (1991a). Periodic limb movements in sleep in community-dwelling elderly. *Sleep, 14*, 496–500.

Ancoli-Israel, S., Kripke, D. F., Klauber, M. R., Mason, W. J., Fell, R., & Kaplan, O. (1991b). Sleep-disordered breathing in community-dwelling elderly. *Sleep, 14*, 486–495.

Angst, J., Vollrath, M., Koch, R., & Dobler-Mikola, A. (1989). The Zurich study. VII. Insomnia: Symptoms, classification and prevalence. *European Archives of Psychiatry and Neurological Science, 238*, 285–293.

Babar, S. I., Enright, P. L., Boyle, P., Foley, D., Sharp, D. S., Petrovitch, H., & Quan, S. F. (2000). Sleep disturbances and their correlates in elderly Japanese American men residing in Hawaii. *Journal of Gerontology: Medical Sciences, 55A*, M406–411.

Babkoff, H., Weller, A., & Lavidor, M. (1996). A comparison of prospective and retrospective assessments of sleep. *Journal of Clinical Epidemiology, 49*, 455–460.

Backhaus, J., Hohagen, F., Voderholzer, U., & Riemann, D. (2001). Long-term effectiveness of a short-term cognitive-behavioral group treatment for primary insomnia. *European Archives of Psychiatry and Clinical Neuroscience, 251*, 35–41.

Bastien, C. H., LeBlanc, M., Carrier, J., & Morin, C. M. (2003). Sleep EEG power spectra, insomnia, and chronic use of benzodiazepines. *Sleep, 26*, 313–317.

Beck, A. T., & Steer, R. A. (1987). *Beck Depression Inventory*. Orlando, FL: Psychological Corporation.

Beck, A. T., Steer, R. A., & Garbin, M. G. (1988). Psychometric properties of the Beck Depression Inventory: Twenty-five years of evaluation. *Clinical Psychology Review, 8*, 77–100.

Bixler, E. O., & Vela-Bueno, A. (1987). Normal sleep: Patterns and mechanisms. *Seminars in Neurology, 7*, 227–235.

Bixler, E. O., Kales, A., Soldatos, C. R., Kales, J. D., & Healey, S. (1979). Prevalence of sleep disorders in the Los Angeles metropolitan area. *American Journal of Psychiatry, 136*, 1257–1262.

Blazer, D. G., Hays, J. C., & Foley, D. J. (1995). Sleep complaints in older adults: A racial comparison. *Journal of Gerontology: Medical Sciences, 50A*, M280–M284.

Bliwise, D. L. (2000). Normal aging. In M. H. Kryger, T. Roth, & W. C. Dement (Eds.), *Principles and practice of sleep medicine* (3rd ed., pp. 26–42). Philadelphia: Saunders.

Bliwise, D. L., Friedman, L., Nekich, J. C., & Yesavage, J. A. (1995). Prediction of outcome in behaviorally based insomnia treatments. *Journal of Behavior Therapy and Experimental Psychiatry, 26*, 17–23.

Bliwise, D. L., King, A. C., & Harris, R. B. (1994). Habitual sleep durations and health in a 50–65 year old population. *Journal of Clinical Epidemiology, 47*, 35–41.

Bonnet, M. H., & Arand, D. L. (1997). Hyperarousal and insomnia. *Sleep Medicine Reviews, 1*, 97–108.

Brabbins, C. J., Dewey, M. E., Copeland, J. R. M., Davidson, I. A., McWilliam, C., Saunders, P., Sharma, V. K., & Sullivan, C. (1993). Insomnia in the elderly: Prevalence, gender differences and relationships with morbidity and mortality. *International Journal of Geriatric Psychiatry, 8*, 473–480.

Broman, J. E., Lundh, L. G., & Hetta, J. (1996). Insufficient sleep in the general population. *Neurophysiologie Clinique, 26*, 30–39.

Brunner, J. A., & Brunner, G. A. (1971). Are voluntarily unlisted telephone subscribers really different? *Journal of Marketing Research, 8*, 121–124.

Campbell, S. S., Gillin, J. C., Kripke, D. F., Erikson, P., & Clopton, P. (1989). Gender differences in the circadian temperature rhythms of healthy elderly subjects: Relationships to sleep quality. *Sleep, 12*, 529–536.

Cannell, C., Groves, R., Magilavy, L., Mathiowetz, N., & Miller, P. (1987). An experimental comparison of telephone and personal health surveys. *Vital Health Statistics, Series 2*. Washington DC: U.S. Government Printing Office.

Carskadon, M. A., Dement, W. C., Mitler, M. M., Guilleminault, C., Zarcone, V. P., & Spiegel, R. (1976). Self-reports versus sleep laboratory findings in 122 drug-free subjects with complaints of chronic insomnia. *American Journal of Psychiatry, 133*, 1382–1388.

Cassidy, D. C. (1992). *Uncertainty: The life and science of Werner Heisenberg*. New York: Freeman.

Chevalier, H., Los, F., Boichut, D., Bianchi, M., Nutt, D. J., Hajak, G., Hetta, J., Hoffmann, G., & Crowe, C. (1999). Evaluation of severe insomnia in the general population: Results of a European multinational survey. *Journal of Psychopharmacology, 13*, S21–24.

Chiu, H. F., Leung, T., Lam, L. C., Wing, Y. K., Chung, D. W., Li, S. W., Chi, I., Law, W. T., & Boey, K. W. (1999). Sleep problems in Chinese elderly in Hong Kong. *Sleep, 22*, 717–726.

Cohen, J. (1987). *Statistical power analysis for the behavioral sciences*. Hillsdale, NJ: Erlbaum.

Cole Information Services. (1999). *Cole Cross Reference Directory: Memphis and Vicinity*. Lincoln, NE: Author.

Corbie-Smith, G., Thomas, S. B., & St. George, D. M. M. (2002). Distrust, race, and research. *Archives of Internal Medicine, 162*, 2458–2463.

Cragg, K., Perlis, M., Aloia, M., Boehmler, J., Millikan, A., Greenblatt, D., & Giles, D. (1999). Questionnaire vs. diary assessments of sleep complaints. *Sleep, 22* (Suppl. 1), S244.

Crawford, S. D., Couper, M. P., & Lamias, M. J. (2001). Web surveys: Perceptions of burden. *Social Science Computer Review, 19,* 146–162.

Cunningham, J. A., Ansara, D., Wild, T. C., Toneatto, T., & Koski-Jannes, A. (1999). What is the price of perfection? The hidden costs of using detailed assessment instruments to measure alcohol consumption. *Journal of Studies on Alcohol, 60,* 756–758.

Davis, K., & Rowland, D. (1983). Uninsured and underserved: Inequities in health care in the United States. *Milbank Memorial Fund Quarterly/Health and Society, 61* (2), 149–176.

Dillman, D. A. (1978). *Mail and telephone surveys: The total design method.* New York: Wiley.

Doi, Y., Minowa, M., Okawa, M., & Uchiyama, M. (1999). Prevalence of sleep disturbance and hypnotic medication use in relation to sociodemographic factors in the general Japanese adult population. *Journal of Epidemiology, 10,* 79–86.

Durrence, H. H., & Lichstein, K. L. (2003). *The sleep of African Americans.* Manuscript submitted for publication.

Edinger, J. D., Fins, A. I., Sullivan, R. J., Jr., Marsh, G. R., Dailey, D. S., Hope, T. V., Young, M., Shaw, E., Carlson, D., & Vasilas, D. (1997). Sleep in the laboratory and sleep at home: Comparisons of older insomniacs and normal sleepers. *Sleep, 20,* 1119–1126.

Espie, C. A. (1991). *The psychological treatment of insomnia.* Chichester, England: Wiley.

Feinberg, I., & Carlson, V. R. (1968). Sleep variables as a function of age in man. *Archives of General Psychiatry, 18,* 239–250.

Ferrara, M., & De Gennaro, L. (2001). How much sleep do we need? *Sleep Medicine Reviews, 5,* 155–179.

Fichten, C. S., Creti, L., Amsel, R., Brender, W., Weinstein, N., & Libman, E. (1995). Poor sleepers who do not complain of insomnia: Myths and realities about psychological and lifestyle characteristics of older good and poor sleepers. *Journal of Behavioral Medicine, 18,* 189–223.

Fichten, C. S., Libman, E., Bailes, S., & Alapin, I. (2000). Characteristics of older adults with insomnia. In K. L. Lichstein & C. M. Morin (Eds.), *Treatment of late-life insomnia* (pp. 37–79). Thousand Oaks, CA: Sage.

Fletcher, J., & Thompson, H. (1974). Telephone directory samples and random telephone number generation. *Journal of Broadcasting, 18,* 187–191.

Foley, D. J., Monjan, A. A., Brown, S. L., Simonsick, E. M., Wallace, R. B., & Blazer, D. G. (1995). Sleep complaints among elderly persons: An epidemiologic study of three communities. *Sleep, 18,* 425–432.

Foley, D. J., Monjan, A. A., Izmirlian, G., Hays, J. C., & Blazer, D. G. (1999). Incidence and remission of insomnia among elderly adults in a biracial cohort. *Sleep, 22* (Suppl. 2), S373–S378.

Ford, D. E., & Kamerow, D. B. (1989). Epidemiologic study of sleep disturbances and psychiatric disorders: An opportunity for prevention? *Journal of the American Medical Association, 262,* 1479–1484.

Frankel, J., & Sharp, L. (1981). Measurement of respondent burden. *Statistical Reporter,* 105–111.

Gallup Organization. (1995). *Sleep in America: 1995.* Princeton, NJ: Author.

Ganguli, M., Reynolds, C. F., & Gilby, J. E. (1996). Prevalence and persistence of sleep complaints in a rural older community sample: The MoVIES project. *Journal of the American Geriatrics Society, 44,* 778–784.

Gislason, R., & Almqvist, M. (1987). Somatic diseases and sleep complaints: An epidemiological study of 3,201 Swedish men. *Acta Medica Scandinavica, 221,* 475–481.

Gislason, T., Reynisdottir, H., Kristbjarnarson, H., & Benediktsdottir, B. (1993). Sleep habits and sleep disturbances among the elderly—An epidemiological survey. *Journal of Internal Medicine, 234,* 31–39.

Gorin, A. A., & Stone, A. A. (2001). Recall biases and cognitive errors in retrospective self-reports: A call for momentary assessments. In A. Baum, T. A. Revenson, & J. E. Singer (Eds.), *Handbook of health psychology* (pp. 405–413). Mahwah, NJ: Lawrence Erlbaum Associates.

Groves, R. M., & Fultz, N. H. (1985). Gender effects among telephone interviewers in a survey of economic attitudes. *Sociological Methods and Research, 14,* 31–52.

Groves, R. M., & Kahn, R. L. (1979). *Surveys by telephone: A national comparison with personal interviews.* New York: Academic Press.

Groves, R. M., Biemer, P. P., Lyberg, L. E., Massey, J. T., Nicholls, W. L. II, & Waksberg, J. (Eds.). (1988). *Telephone survey methodology.* New York: Wiley.

Habte-Gabr, E., Wallace, R. B., Colsher, P. L., Hulbert, J. R., White, L. R., & Smith, I. M. (1991). Sleep patterns in rural elders: Demographic, health, and psychobehavioral correlates. *Journal of Clinical Epidemiology, 44,* 5–13.

Hauri, P. J. (1997). Can we mix behavioral therapy with hypnotics when treating insomniacs? *Sleep, 20,* 1111–1118.

Haynes, S. N., Adams, A. E., West, S., Kamens, L., & Safranek, R. (1982). The stimulus control paradigm in sleep-onset insomnia: A multimethod assessment. *Journal of Psychosomatic Research, 26,* 333–339.

Hays, W. L. (1963). *Statistics.* New York: Holt, Rinehart and Winston.

Henderson, S., Jorm, A. F., Scott, L. R., Mackinnon, A. J., Christensen, H., & Korten, A. E. (1995). Insomnia in the elderly: Its prevalence and correlates in the general population. *Medical Journal of Australia, 162,* 22–24.

Herscovitch, J., & Broughton, R. (1981). Sensitivity of the Stanford Sleepiness Scale to the effects of cumulative partial sleep deprivation and recovery oversleeping. *Sleep, 4,* 83–92.

Hicks, R. A., Lucero-Gorman, K., Bautista, J., & Hicks, G. J. (1999). Ethnicity, sleep duration, and sleep satisfaction. *Perceptual and Motor Skills, 88,* 234–235.

Hoddes, E., Zarcone, V., Smythe, H., Phillips, R., & Dement, W. C. (1973). Quantification of sleepiness: A new approach. *Psychophysiology, 10,* 431–436.

Hoelscher, T. J., Ware, J. C., & Bond, T. (1993). Initial validation of the Insomnia Impact Scale. *Sleep Research, 22,* 149.

Huitema, B. E. (1980). *The analysis of covariance and alternatives.* New York: Wiley.

Husby, R., & Lingjaerde, O. (1990). Prevalence of reported sleeplessness in northern Norway in relation to sex, age and season. *Acta Psychiatrica Scandinavica, 81,* 542–547.

Janson, C., Gislason, T., De Backer, W., Plaschke, P., Bjornsson, E., Hetta, J., Kristbjarnason, H., Vermeire, P., & Boman, G. (1995). Prevalence of sleep disturbances among young adults in three European countries. *Sleep, 18,* 589–597.

Jean-Louis, G., Kripke, D. F., & Ancoli-Israel, S. (2000). Sleep and quality of well-being. *Sleep, 23,* 1115–1121.

Jean-Louis, G., Magai, C. M., Cohen, C. I., Zizi, F., von Gizycki, H., DiPalma, J., & Casimir, G. J. (2001). Ethnic differences in self-reported sleep problems in older adults. *Sleep, 24,* 926–933.

Johns, M. W. (1991). A new method for measuring daytime sleepiness: The Epworth sleepiness scale. *Sleep, 14,* 540–545.

Johns, M. W. (1994). Sleepiness in different situations measured by the Epworth Sleepiness Scale. *Sleep, 17,* 703–710.

Johns, M., & Hocking, B. (1997). Daytime sleepiness and sleep habits of Australian workers. *Sleep, 20,* 844–849.

Jones, W., Jr., & Rene, A. A. (1994). Barriers to health services utilization and African Americans. In I. L. Livingston (Ed.), *Handbook of Black American health* (pp. 378–386). Westport, CT: Greenwood Press.

Kahn, K., Pearson, M. L., Harrison, E. R., Desmond, K. A., Rogers, W. H., Rubenstein, L. V., Brook, R. H., & Keeler, E. B. (1994). Health care for Black and poor hospitalized Medicare patients. *Journal of the American Medical Association, 271,* 1169–1174.

Kales, A., & Kales, J. D. (1984). *Evaluation and treatment of insomnia.* New York: Oxford University Press.

Karacan, I., Thornby, J. I., & Williams, R. L. (1983). Sleep disturbance: A community survey. In C. Guilleminault & E. Lugaresi (Eds.), *Sleep/wake disorders: Natural history, epidemiology, and long-term evolution* (pp. 37–60). New York: Raven Press.

Karacan, I., Thornby, J. I., Anch, M., Holzer, C. E., Warheit, G. J., Schwab, J. J., & Williams, R. L. (1976). Prevalence of sleep disturbance in a primarily urban Florida county. *Social Science and Medicine, 10,* 239–244.

Kim, K., Uchiyama, M., Okawa, M., Liu, X., & Ogihara, R. (2000). An epidemiological study of insomnia among the Japanese general population. *Sleep, 23,* 41–47.

Klink, M., & Quan, S. F. (1987). Prevalence of reported sleep disturbances in a general adult population and their relationship to obstructive airways diseases. *Chest, 91,* 540–546.

Korotitsch, W. J., & Nelson-Gray, R. O. (1999). An overview of self-monitoring research in assessment and treatment. *Psychological Assessment, 11,* 415–425.

Kripke, D. F., Ancoli-Israel, S., Klauber, M. R., Wingard, D. L., Mason, W. J., & Mullaney, D. J. (1997). Prevalence of sleep-disordered breathing in ages 40–64 years: A population-based survey. *Sleep, 20,* 65–76.

Kripke, D. F., Brunner, R., Freeman, R., Hendrix, S. L., Jackson, R. D., Masaki, K., & Carter, R. A. (2001). Sleep complaints of postmenopausal women. *Clinical Journal of Women's Health, 1,* 244–252

Krupp, L. B., LaRocca, N. G., Muir-Nash, J., & Steinberg, A. D. (1989). The Fatigue Severity Scale: Application to patients with multiple sclerosis and systemic lupus erythematosus. *Archives of Neurology, 46,* 1121–1123.

Kupfer, D. J., & Reynolds, C. F. III. (1983). A critical review of sleep and its disorders from a developmental perspective. *Psychiatric Developments, 4,* 367–386.

Lack, L., Miller, W., & Turner, D. (1988). A survey of sleeping difficulties in an Australian population. *Community Health Studies, 12,* 200–207.

Lamberg, L. (2003). Illness, not age itself, most often the trigger of sleep problems in older adults. *Journal of the American Medical Association, 290,* 319–323.

Leger, D., Guilleminault, C., Dreyfus, J. P., Delahaye, C., & Paillard, M. (2000). Prevalence of insomnia in a survey of 12,778 adults in France. *Journal of Sleep Research, 9,* 35–42.

Libman, E., Fichten, C. S., Bailes, S., & Amsel, R. (2000). Sleep questionnaire versus sleep diary: Which measure is better? *International Journal of Rehabilitation and Health, 5,* 205–209.

Lichstein, K. L. (1997). A general index of self-reported sleep: The sleep quotient. *Behaviour Research and Therapy, 35,* 1133–1137.

Lichstein, K. L. (2000). Secondary insomnia. In K. L. Lichstein & C. M. Morin (Eds.), *Treatment of late-life insomnia* (pp. 297–319). Thousand Oaks, CA: Sage.

Lichstein, K. L., Durrence, H. H., Riedel, B. W., & Bayen, U. J. (2001). Primary versus secondary insomnia in older adults: Subjective sleep and daytime functioning. *Psychology and Aging, 16,* 264–271.

Lichstein, K. L., Durrence, H. H., Taylor, D. J., Bush, A. J., & Riedel, B. W. (2003). Quantitative criteria for insomnia. *Behaviour Research and Therapy, 41,* 427–445.

Lichstein, K. L., Means, M. K., Noe, S. L., & Aguillard, R. N. (1997). Fatigue and sleep disorders. *Behaviour Research and Therapy, 35,* 733–740.

Lichstein, K. L., Riedel, B. W., & Means, M. K. (1999). Psychological treatment of late-life insomnia. In R. Schulz, G. Maddox, & M. P. Lawton (Eds.), *Annual review of gerontology and geriatrics, Vol. 18, Focus on interventions research with older adults* (pp. 74–110). New York: Springer.

Lichstein, K. L., Riedel, B. W., Wilson, N. M., Lester, K. W., & Aguillard, R. N. (2001). Relaxation and sleep compression for late-life insomnia: A placebo-controlled trial. *Journal of Consulting and Clinical Psychology, 69,* 227–239.

Liljenberg, B., Almqvist, M., Hetta, J., Roos, B., & Agren, H. (1988). The prevalence of insomnia: The importance of operationally defined criteria. *Annals of Clinical Research, 20,* 393–398.

Liljenberg, B., Almqvist, M., Hetta, J., Roos, B., & Agren, H. (1989). The prevalence of insomnia in adulthood. *European Journal of Psychiatry, 3,* 5–12.

Livingston, I. L. (Ed.). (1994). *Handbook of Black American health.* Westport, CT: Greenwood Press.

Macera, C. A., Armstead, C. A., & Anderson, N. B. (2001). Sociocultural influences on health. In A. Baum, T. A. Revenson, & J. E. Singer (Eds.), *Handbook of health psychology* (pp. 427–440). Mahwah, NJ: Lawrence Erlbaum Associates.

Maggi, S., Langlois, J. A., Minicuci, N., Grigoletto, F., Pavan, M., Foley, D. J., & Enzi, G. (1998). Sleep complaints in community-dwelling older persons: Prevalence, associated factors, and reported causes. *Journal of the American Geriatrics Society, 46,* 161–168.

Mathews, A. (1997). Information processing biases in emotional disorders. In D. M. Clark & C. G. Fairburn (Eds.), *Science and practice of cognitive behaviour therapy* (pp. 47–66). Oxford: Oxford University Press.

Maxwell, S. E., & Delaney, H. D. (1990). *Designing experiments and analyzing data: A model comparison perspective.* Belmont, CA: Wadsworth.

Means, M. K., Lichstein, K. L., Epperson, M. T., & Johnson, C. T. (2000). Relaxation therapy for insomnia: Nighttime and day time effects. *Behaviour Research and Therapy, 38,* 665–678.

Mellinger, G. D., Balter, M. B., & Uhlenhuth, E. H. (1985). Insomnia and its treatment: Prevalence and correlates. *Archives of General Psychiatry, 42,* 225–232.

Middelkoop, H. A. M., Smilde-van den Doel, D. A., Neven, A. K., Kamphuisen, H. A. C., & Springer, C. P. (1996). Subjective sleep characteristics of 1485 males and females aged 50–93: Effects of sex and age, and factors related to self-evaluated quality of sleep. *Journal of Gerontology, 51A,* M108–115.

Morgan, K. (2000). Sleep and aging. In K. L. Lichstein & C. M. Morin (Eds.), *Treatment of late-life insomnia* (pp. 3–36). Thousand Oaks, CA: Sage.

Morgan, K., Dallosso, H., Ebrahim, S., Arie, T., & Fentem, P. H. (1988). Characteristics of subjective insomnia in the elderly living at home. *Age and Ageing, 17,* 1–7.

Morin, C. M. (1993). *Insomnia: Psychological assessment and management.* New York: Guilford.

Morin, C. M., & Azrin, N. H. (1988). Behavioral and cognitive treatments of geriatric insomnia. *Journal of Consulting and Clinical Psychology, 56,* 748–753.

Morin, C. M., & Gramling, S. E. (1989). Sleep patterns and aging: Comparison of older adults with and without insomnia complaints. *Psychology and Aging, 4,* 290–294.

Morin, C. M., Kowatch, R. A., Barry, T., & Walton, E. (1993). Cognitive-behavior therapy for late-life insomnia. *Journal of Consulting and Clinical Psychology, 61,* 137–146.

Mulry-Liggan, M. H. (1983). A comparison of a RDD survey and the current population survey. *Proceedings of the Section on Survey Research Methods, American Statistical Association,* 231–233.

Murrell, N. L., Smith, R., Gill, G., & Oxley, G. (1996). Racism and health care access: A dialogue with childbearing women. *Health Care for Women International, 17,* 149–159.

National Sleep Foundation. (2002). *2002 Sleep in America poll.* Washington, DC: Author.

Newman, A. B., Enright, P. L., Manolio, T. A., Haponik, E. F., & Wahl, P. W. (1997). Sleep disturbance, psychosocial correlates, and cardiovascular disease in 5201 older adults: The cardiovascular health study. *Journal of the American Geriatrics Society, 45,* 1–7.

Ohayon, M. (1996). Epidemiological study on insomnia in the general population. *Sleep, 19,* S7–S15.

Ohayon, M. M. (2002). Epidemiology of insomnia: What we know and what we still need to learn. *Sleep Medicine Reviews, 6,* 97–111.

Ohayon, M. M., Caulet, M., & Guilleminault, C. (1997). How a general population perceives its sleep and how this relates to the complaint of insomnia. *Sleep, 20,* 715–723.

Ohayon, M. M., Caulet, M., Priest, R. G., & Guilleminault, C. (1997). DSM-IV and ICSD–90 insomnia symptoms and sleep dissatisfaction. *British Journal of Psychiatry, 171,* 382–388.

Olson, L. G. (1996). A community survey of insomnia in Newcastle. *Australian and New Zealand Journal of Public Health, 20,* 655–657.

Partinen, M., Kaprio, J., Koskenvuo, M., & Langinvainio, H. (1983). Sleeping habits, sleep quality, and use of sleeping pills: A population study of 31,140 adults in Finland. In C. Guilleminault & E. Lugaresi (Eds.), *Sleep/wake disorders: Natural history, epidemiology, and long-term evolution* (pp. 29–35). New York: Raven Press.

Pressman, M. R., & Fry, J. M. (1989). Relationship of autonomic nervous system activity to daytime sleepiness and prior sleep. *Sleep, 12,* 239–245.

Profant, J., Ancoli-Israel, S., & Dimsdale, J. E. (2002). Are there ethnic differences in sleep architecture? *American Journal of Human Biology, 14,* 321–326.

Quera-Salva, M. A., Orluc, A., Goldenberg, F., & Guilleminault, C. (1991). Insomnia and the use of hypnotics: Study of a French population. *Sleep, 14,* 386–391.

Qureshi, A. I., Giles, W. H., Croft, J. B., & Bliwise, D. L. (1997). Habitual sleep patterns and risk for stroke and coronary heart disease: A 10-year follow-up from NHANES I. *Neurology, 48,* 904–911.

Rao, U., Poland, R. E., Lutchmansingh, P., Ott, G. E., McCracken, J. T., & Keh-Ming, L. (1999). Relationship between ethnicity and sleep patterns in normal controls: Implications for psychopathology and treatment. *Journal of Psychiatric Research, 33,* 419–426.

Riedel, B. W., & Lichstein, K. L. (2000). Insomnia and daytime functioning. *Sleep Medicine Reviews, 4,* 277–298.

Roberts, R. E., Shema, S. J., & Kaplan, G. A. (1999). Prospective data on sleep complaints and associated risk factors in an older cohort. *Psychosomatic Medicine, 61,* 188–196.

Rocha, F. L., Uchoa, E., Guerra, H. L., Firmo, J. O. A., Vidigal, P. G., & Lima-Costa, M. F. (2002). Prevalence of sleep complaints and associated factors in community-dwelling older people in Brazil: The Bambui health and ageing study (BHAS). *Sleep Medicine, 3,* 231–238.

Roth, T., & Ancoli-Israel, S. (1999). Daytime consequences and correlates of insomnia in the United States: Results of the 1991 National Sleep Foundation Survey. II. *Sleep, 22* (Suppl. 2), S354–S358.

Schoenborn, C. A. (1986). Health habits of U.S. adults, 1985: The "Alameda 7" revisited. *Public Health Reports, 101,* 571–580.

Schwartz, J. E., Jandorf, L., & Krupp, L. B. (1993). The measurement of fatigue: A new instrument. *Journal of Psychosomatic Research, 37,* 753–762.

Seppala, M., Hyyppa, M. T., Impivaara, O., Knuts, L. R., & Sourander, L. (1997). Subjective quality of sleep and use of hypnotics in an elderly urban population. *Aging: Clinical and Experimental Research, 9,* 327–334.

Shadish, W. R., Cook, T. D., & Campbell, D. T. (2002). *Experimental and quasi-experimental designs for generalized causal inference.* Boston: Houghton Mifflin.

Shadish, W. R., Robinson, L. A., & Lu, C. (1997). *ES: A computer program and manual for effect size calculation.* Memphis, TN: University of Memphis.

Shavers-Hornaday, V. L., Lynch, C. F., Burmeister, L. F., & Torner, J. C. (1997). Why are African Americans under-represented in medical research studies? Impediments to participation. *Ethnicity and Health, 2,* 31–45.

Shealy, R. C., Lowe, J. D., & Ritzler, B. A. (1980). Sleep onset insomnia: Personality characteristics and treatment outcome. *Journal of Consulting and Clinical Psychology, 48,* 659–661.

Sinharay, S., Stern, H. S., & Russell, D. (2001). The use of multiple imputation for the analysis of missing data. *Psychological Methods, 6,* 317–329.

Snowden, L. R. (2001). Barriers to effective mental health services for African Americans. *Mental Health Services Research, 3,* 181–187.

Spielberger, C. D., Gorsuch, R. L., Lushene, R., Vagg, P. R., & Jacobs, G. A. (1983). *State-Trait Anxiety Inventory (Form Y).* Palo Alto, CA: Consulting Psychologists Press.

Stepnowsky, C. J., Jr., Moore, P. J., & Dimsdale, J. E. (2003). Effect of ethnicity on sleep: Complexities for epidemiologic research. *Sleep, 26,* 329–332.

Sutton, D. A., Moldofsky, H., & Badley, E. M. (2001). Insomnia and health problems in Canadians. *Sleep, 24,* 665–670.

Tanaka-Matsumi, J., & Kameoka, V. A. (1986). Reliabilities and concurrent validities of popular self-report measures of depression, anxiety, and social desirability. *Journal of Consulting and Clinical Psychology, 54,* 328–333.

Tennessee Department of Health. (2000). *Community health status, Shelby County, Tennessee.* Retrieved 20 March 2002 from http://www.communityhealth.hrsa.gov/Documents/V-TN/CHSI-V-47-157-TN-Shelby.pdf

U.S. Census Bureau. (2000). *Census 2000.* http://www.census.gov.

U.S. Population Reference Bureau. (2000). *2000 United States Population Data Sheet.* Retrieved 20 March 2002 from http://www.prb.org/content/navigationmenu/other_reports/2000-2002/2000_United_States_Population_Data_Sheet.htm#section6

Voderholzer, U., Al-Shajlawi, A., Weske, G., Feige, B., & Riemann, D. (2003). Are there gender differences in objective and subjective sleep measures? A study of insomniacs and healthy controls. *Depression and Anxiety, 17,* 162–172.

Weaver, C. N., Holmes, S. L., & Glenn, N. D. (1975). Some characteristics of inaccessible respondents in a telephone survey. *Journal of Applied Psychology, 60,* 260–262.

Webb, W. B. (1965). Sleep characteristics of human subjects. *Bulletin of the British Psychological Society, 18,* 1–10.

Welstein, L., Dement, W. C., Redington, D., Guilleminault, C., & Mitler, M. M. (1983). Insomnia in the San Francisco Bay Area: A telephone survey. *Sleep/wake disorders: Natural history, epidemiology, and long-term evolution* (pp. 73–85). New York: Raven Press.

Weyerer, S., & Dilling, H. (1991). Prevalence and treatment of insomnia in the community: Results from the Upper Bavarian field study. *Sleep, 14,* 392–398.

Williams, R. L., Karacan, I., & Hursch, C. J. (1974). *Electroencephalography (EEG) of human sleep: Clinical applications.* New York: Wiley.

Windholz, G. (1997). Ivan P. Pavlov: An overview of his life and psychological work. *American Psychologist, 52,* 941–946.

Winer, B. J. (1971). *Statistical principles in experimental design* (2nd ed.). New York: McGraw-Hill.

Winkleby, M. A., Jatulis, D. E., Frank, E., & Fortmann, S. P. (1992). Socioeconomic status and health: How education, income, and occupation contribute to risk factors for cardiovascular disease. *American Journal of Public Health, 82,* 816–820.

Wohlgemuth, W. K., Edinger, J. D., Fins, A. I., & Sullivan, R. J. (1999). How many nights are enough? The short-term stability of sleep parameters in elderly insomniacs and normal sleepers. *Psychophysiology, 36,* 233–244.

World Health Organization. (1992). *International statistical classification of diseases and related health problems,* 10th rev. Geneva: Author.

Author Index

229

Subject Index